# ABC OF ADOLESCENCF

Edited by

## RUSSELL VINER

*Consultant in adolescent medicine at University College London Hospitals NHS Foundation Trust*
*tal NHS Trust*

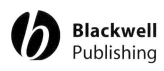

Blackwell Publishing, Inc., 350 Main Street, Malden, Massachusetts 02148-5020, USA
Blackwell Publishing Ltd, 9600 Garsington Road, Oxford OX4 2DQ, UK
Blackwell Publishing Asia Pty Ltd, 550 Swanston Street, Carlton, Victoria 3053, Australia

First published 2005

**Library of Congress Cataloging-in-Publication Data**
ABC of adolescence/edited by Russell Viner.
          p.   ;   cm.
    Includes bibliographical references and index.
    ISBN-13: 978-0-7279-1574-0
    ISBN-10: 0-7279-1574-6
  1.   Adolescent medicine. 2.   Adolescence.
    [DNLM: 1. Adolescent medicine. WS 460 A134 2005] I. Viner, Russell.

  RJ550.A23 2005
  616′.00835—dc22

                                                              2005012252

ISBN-13: 978 0 7279 1574 0
ISBN-10: 0 7279 1574 6

A catalogue record for this title is available from the British Library

Set by BMJ Electronic Production
Printed and bound in Spain by GraphyCems, Navarra

Commissioning Editor: Eleanor Lines
Senior Technical Editor: Julia Thompson
Development Editors: Sally Carter, Nick Morgan
Production Controller: Debbie Wyer

For further information on Blackwell Publishing, visit our website:
http://www.blackwellpublishing.com

The publisher's policy is to use permanent paper from mills that operate a sustainable forestry
policy, and which has been manufactured from pulp processed using acid-free and elementary
chlorine-free practices. Furthermore, the publisher ensures that the text paper and cover board
used have met acceptable environmental accreditation standards.

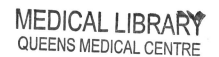

# Contents

# Contributors

**Yvonne Bonomo**
Senior lecturer, paediatrics department, University of Melbourne, Parkville, Australia

**Robert Booy**
Epidemiologist and professor of child health, Barts and the London School of Medicine and Dentistry Medical School

**Deborah Christie**
Consultant clinical psychologist, Middlesex Adolescence Unit, University College London Hospitals NHS Foundation Trust, London

**Eric Fombonne**
Canada Research Chair in child psychiatry, Professor of Psychiatry, McGill University, and Director of the Department of Psychiatry at the Montreal Children's Hospital

**Keith Hawton**
Professor of psychiatry and director of the Centre for Suicide Research, University of Oxford, and consultant psychiatrist, Oxfordshire Mental Healthcare Trust, Warneford Hospital, Oxford

**Anthony James**
Consultant in adolescent psychiatry, Highfield Adolescent Unit, Oxfordshire Mental Healthcare Trust, Warneford Hospital, Oxford

**Vic Larcher**
Consultant paediatrician, Barts and the London NHS Trust

**Aidan Macfarlane**
Independent international consultant in the strategic planning of child and adolescent health services, Oxford, UK

**Ann McPherson**
Department of Primary Care, University of Oxford

**Pierre-André Michaud**
Medical director of the multidisciplinary adolescent unit, Centre Hospitalier Universitaire Vaudois, Lausanne, Switzerland

**Dasha Nicholls**
Consultant child and adolescent psychiatrist, Feeding and Eating Disorders Service, Great Ormond Street Hospital, London

**Jenny Proimos**
Consultant in adolescent medicine, Centre for Adolescent Health, Royal Children's Hospital, Melbourne, Australia

**Susan Sawyer**
Professor and director, Centre for Adolescent Health, Royal Children's Hospital, Melbourne, Australia

**John Tripp**
Consultant paediatrician and senior lecturer in child health, Peninsula Medical School, Universities of Exeter and Plymouth

**Russell Viner**
Consultant in adolescent medicine, University College London Hospitals NHS Foundation Trust and Great Ormond Street Hospital NHS Trust

**Michele Yeo**
Adolescent physician, Centre for Adolescent Health, Royal Children's Hospital, Melbourne, Australia

# Preface

Adolescence, the period between childhood and adulthood, is increasingly recognised as a life period that poses specific challenges for treating illness and promoting health. In working with adolescents, all aspects of clinical medicine and public health are played out against a background of rapid physical, psychological, and social developmental changes. Working with young people is usually extremely rewarding—and often great fun.

Many prevalent assumptions about the health of young people are incorrect. Although young people are generally thought to be healthy, most of them visit their general practitioner each year, and in areas such as sexually transmitted infections, depression, obesity, and eating disorders, problems are growing rather than diminishing. Indeed, adolescents seem to be the age group whose health has improved least over the past 40 years.

Young people and health professionals often feel that communication between them is problematic. Indeed, working with young people is the only time in clinical practice when health professionals do not deal directly with adults, either as parents or as patients.

Given the right information and skills, practising medicine with young people can be extremely rewarding and fruitful. The aim of this ABC series is to provide a basic overview of the subject for all who work with adolescents. The first half of the book provides a general developmental, ethical and legal, and health promotion framework in which to place working with young people, as well as pointers for caring for adolescents in primary and secondary care. The second half of the book focuses on some of the most important issues in adolescent health, including mental health, sexual health, drug and alcohol problems, fatigue, and eating disorders and obesity.

I would like to thank Aidan Macfarlane for starting this project before passing it on to me, and to particularly thank George Patton and Susan Sawyer from the Centre for Adolescent Health in Melbourne for supporting my work in adolescent health. Thanks also go to my colleagues from Australia, Switzerland, and Canada, as well as those from the United Kingdom for their work in contributing chapters. Most thanks, however, go to the BMJ editors, Eleanor Lines and Julia Thompson, for keeping me on the straight and narrow when other commitments and clinical constraints threatened to delay the project.

Russell Viner
2005

# 1 Adolescent development

Deborah Christie, Russell Viner

In the care of adolescent patients, all aspects of clinical medicine are played out against a background of rapid physical, psychological, and social developmental changes. These changes produce specific disease patterns, unusual presentations of symptoms, and above all, unique communication and management challenges. This can make working with adolescents difficult. However, with the right skills, practising medicine with young people can be rewarding and fruitful. These skills are needed by everyone who works with young people in the course of their work.

As a young person enters adolescence, their parents are still largely responsible for all aspects of their health. By the end of adolescence, health issues will be almost entirely the responsibility of the young person. The challenge is to maintain an effective clinical relationship while the health responsibilities transfer from the parents to the young person.

Specialised clinical communication skills are needed to take an accurate history, bearing in mind new life domains not applicable to children (sex and drugs) and adding communication and engagement of the family to the standard adult consultation. Physical examinations of adolescents require consideration of privacy and personal integrity as well as requiring additional skills such as pubertal assessment. For effective treatment of illness in adolescence, doctors need to know about adolescent development if they are to manage adeptly issues of adherence (compliance), identity, consent and confidentiality, and relationships between young people and their families. Evidence from randomised controlled trials clearly shows that such skills can be developed and practised effectively in primary care.

## Developmental tasks

During adolescence young people will negotiate puberty and the completion of growth, take on sexually dimorphic body shape, develop new cognitive skills (including abstract thinking capacities), develop a clearer sense of personal and sexual identity, and develop a degree of emotional, personal, and financial independence from their parents.

**Adolescence is increasingly recognised as a life period that poses specific challenges for treating disease and promoting health**

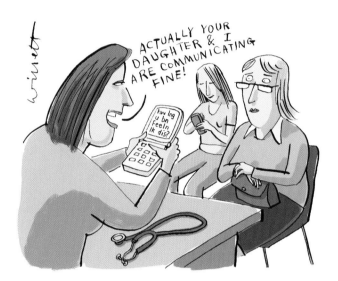

### The primary challenges of adolescence

- The achievement of biological and sexual maturation
- The development of personal identity
- The development of intimate sexual relationships with an appropriate peer
- Establishment of independence and autonomy in the context of the sociocultural environment

### Developmental tasks of adolescence

|  | **Biological** | **Psychological** | **Social** |
|---|---|---|---|
| Early adolescence | Early puberty (girls: breast bud and pubic hair development, start of growth spurt; boys: testicular enlargement, start of genital growth) | Concrete thinking but early moral concepts; progression of sexual identity development (sexual orientation); possible homosexual peer interest; reassessment of body image | Emotional separation from parents; start of strong peer identification; early exploratory behaviours (smoking, violence) |
| Mid-adolescence | Girls: mid-late puberty and end of growth spurt; menarche; development of female body shape with fat deposition<br>Boys: mid-puberty, spermarche and nocturnal emissions; voice breaks; start of growth spurt | Abstract thinking, but self still seen as "bullet proof"; growing verbal abilities; identification of law with morality; start of fervent ideology (religious, political) | Emotional separation from parents; strong peer identification; increased health risk (smoking, alcohol, etc); heterosexual peer interest; early vocational plans |
| Late adolescence | Boys: end of puberty; continued increase in muscle bulk and body hair | Complex abstract thinking; identification of difference between law and morality; increased impulse control; further development of personal identify; further development or rejection of religious and political ideology | Development of social autonomy; intimate relationships; development of vocational capability and financial independence |

*Adapted from McIntosh N, Helms P, Smyth R, eds. *Forfar and Arneil's textbook of paediatrics.* 6th ed. Edinburgh: Churchill Livingstone, 2003:1757-68.

All clinical interactions with adolescents must be seen against this dynamic background of development. Issues around the management of chronic illness, for example, can be quite different with a 13 year old boy in very early puberty who has poorly developed abstract thinking compared with a 16 year old girl who is sexually mature, at final height, and has well developed adult cognitive skills.

## Psychosocial development

The physical changes that signal the start of adolescence occur alongside psychological and social changes that mark this period as a critical stage in becoming an adult. Several models or theories have placed adolescence in a period of human development from birth to death. Most of these are "stage" models—with each stage completed before the individual moves on to the next.

Each model identifies a different set of "tasks" as defining adolescence. Freud focused on psychosexual development, seeing adolescence as a recapitulation of the development of sexual awareness in infancy. Piaget focused on cognitive development, seeing the development of abstract thinking abilities as making possible the transition to independent adult functioning. Most recently, Erikson identified the tensions around the development of personal identity as central to the notion of adolescence. A more useful model is the biopsychosocial approach, which acknowledges that adolescence has biological (puberty and sexual development) as well as psychological and social elements.

A criticism of many of the models describing the adolescent period is their failure to acknowledge explicitly that the young person is in a "system." Their position in the system is determined by their relationships with different parts of the system and mediated by both external and internal demands (or tasks).

Internal physical and psychological changes interact with the external or social changes. The successful achievement and negotiation of the different tasks are therefore interdependent and rely on each other occurring at the appropriate time. When these challenges intersect with health or illness, they produce unique communication and management challenges, particularly around risk taking behaviours and adherence to medical advice or regimens.

### Psychological changes
In early adolescence, young people gradually begin to develop abstract thinking—that is, the ability to use internal symbols or images to represent reality. In contrast to the more childish concrete thinking—where objects have to represent "things" or "ideas" for solving problems—abstract thinking enables us to think hypothetically about the future and assess multiple outcomes. You need to know whether the young person you are communicating with has a poorly or well developed capacity for abstract thinking, as this capacity is essential if he or she is to give informed consent to treatment and be able to manage chronic illness regimens independently.

It is important to recognise the interactions of psychological developments with puberty, particularly in the context of a developing sense of sexuality and body image. Body image and self esteem are vulnerable to differences in the timing of puberty among peers and to the physical effects of chronic illnesses.

### Social changes
Adolescence is usually described as a period in which independence is achieved. It is more accurate, however, to talk about a change in the balance of independence and

> **Whereas puberty and cognitive development are largely biologically determined, the greater part of psychological and social development will depend on environmental and sociocultural influences. In non-Western cultures, the social and psychological domains may be markedly truncated**

> **It may be hard to remember our childhood accurately, but few people forget their adolescence**

---

**The challenges for young people**

- Challenging authority
- Taking risks
- Experimenting with drugs, alcohol, and sex
- Challenging the moral and social structure of society
- Demanding rights
- Taking responsibility for self and others
- Seeking spiritual paths (organised or cult religions)
- Getting a job
- Changing schools and educational environment
- Developing relationships
- Understanding sexuality
- Renegotiating rules at home

---

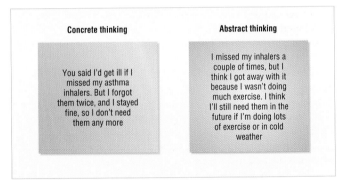

Examples of concrete and abstract thinking by young people in clinical interactions

---

**Psychological effects of timing of puberty**

|  | Early puberty | Late puberty |
|---|---|---|
| Biological | Taller than peers but may end up short | Short stature but later should achieve normal height; osteoporosis |
| Psychological | Psychological effects positive in boys (higher self esteem), negative in girls (low self esteem) | Low self esteem in boys; no major problems in girls |
| Social | Different from peers; treated as adolescent while still a child | Treated by adults and peers as less mature than real age; difficulty in separating from parents and in getting work |

dependence with other parts of the young person's system (parents, peers, community, and even health professionals). The timing of these changes depends on the different social and cultural expectations of the environment in which the young person lives.

As adolescents start to redefine themselves in relation to others, they begin to move to a position where they define other people in relation to themselves. This way of thinking about oneself means that it can be hard to understand the impact of behaviour on others or to feel concern for how others might be affected by behaviour. Knowledge that has been "handed down" by adults is given little value. Adolescents may also strongly believe that no other person can have a clear understanding of how a young person feels.

# Physical development

Psychological development occurs against a background of rapid physical change, including puberty, the pubertal growth spurt, and accompanying maturational changes in other organ systems. Both boys and girls pass through identifiable stages of development of secondary sex characteristics (Tanner stages).

The change from prepuberty to full reproductive capacity may take as little as 18 months or as long as five years. At age 13 years, boys can manifest the entire range. Although girls seem to enter puberty long before boys, the earliest sign in boys (increasing testicular volume), begins at a mean age of 12 years, only six months after girls development breast buds (the first sign of puberty).

Girls also seem considerably more developed earlier as the female growth spurt occurs early in puberty (mean age 11-12 years) compared with later in puberty in boys (mean age 14 years).

The defining event of puberty in girls is menarche. The mean age at menarche showed a substantial decline in most developed countries through the first half of the 20th century, stabilising in the 1960s in most countries at around 13 years for white girls and 12.5 years for black girls.

The commonest clinical concerns about puberty are delayed puberty and short stature, particularly in boys. The 97th centile for developing increased testicular volume ($\geq 4$ ml) is 14 years. Thus about 2% of boys will still be prepubertal (and therefore short) at 14-15 years.

This can be quite distressing but is almost always a normal variant (constitutional delay of puberty and growth) that is often familial. By the time most boys present to their doctor, they will have early signs of testicular enlargement, which is easily assessed using an orchidometer.

Boys aged 15 or over with a testicular volume of 4 ml or more can be reassured that puberty is beginning. Those with no signs of puberty by age 15 should be referred to a paediatric endocrinologist for further investigation.

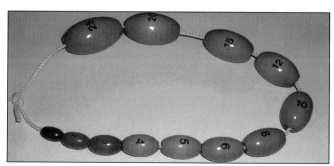

The Prader orchidometer is used for assessing testicular development: 1-3 ml for prepuberty; 4 ml for entering puberty; 8 ml and 10 ml for mid-puberty; and 15 ml to 25 ml for full puberty

**As the ability to think in the abstract develops, it interacts with adolescents' sense of uniqueness to create an awareness of outcomes for others but a belief in personal invulnerability—being "bullet proof." This belief can lead young people to take substantial risks in terms of substance misuse, personal safety, or adherence to treatment, believing that negative outcomes will not apply to them**

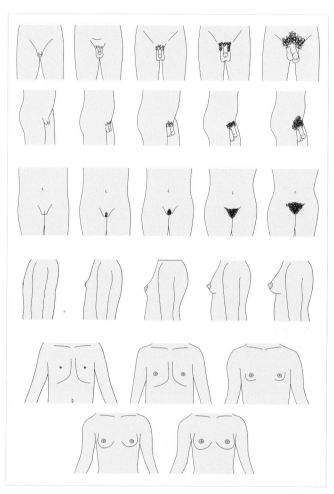

Stages of development of secondary sex characteristics in boys and girls

**Causes of delayed and early puberty**

**Delay in puberty**
- Constitutional delay of growth and puberty (boys)
- Poor nutrition
- Chronic illness
- Eating disorder
- Severe psychosocial stress
- Disorder of hypothalamic-pituitary-gonadal axis

**Early puberty**
- Familial
- Obesity (girls)
- Benign normal variants of pubertal timing: isolated thelarche (early breast development), premature adrenarche (early pubic hair development)
- Abnormalities of the central nervous system that disrupt the hypothalamic-pituitary-gonadal axis
- Gonadotrophin independent "precocious pseudopuberty"

# Communicating with adolescents

Many adolescents and health professionals feel that communication between young people and medical professionals is often highly problematic. Working with young people is the only time in clinical practice when doctors do not deal directly with adults. Adult medicine consists of adult clinicians communicating with other adults, who share largely similar social values and norms about health, even taking account of cultural differences. In paediatrics, professionals negotiate treatment decisions with the parents, with children's participation obtained by explanation and parental authority.

In contrast, in consultations with adolescents, we are faced with the challenge of communicating with a personality undergoing rapid psychological and social changes who may not share an adult's understanding of society or adult cognitive abilities to decide between treatment alternatives in the light of future risks to health. The many versions of "youth culture" that coexist in our increasingly multicultural and ethnically diverse society reinforce this challenge.

Many doctors are not comfortable dealing with adolescents, and general practice studies show that teenagers receive shorter average consultation times from their family doctors than do children or adults. Fortunately, doctors can improve their clinical and communication skills with adolescents through training in adolescent development and in the health needs of adolescents.

## Further reading and resources

- Neinstein LS. *Adolescent health care: a practical guide.* 4th ed. Baltimore: Williams and Wilkins, 2002.
- Strasburger VC, Brown RT. *Adolescent medicine: a practical guide.* 2nd ed. Philadelphia: Lippincott-Raven, 1998.
- *Bridging the gaps: healthcare for adolescents.* (Report of the joint working party on adolescent health of the royal medical and nursing colleges of the UK.) London: Royal College of Paediatrics and Child Health, 2003.
- www.euteach.com and www.adolescenthealth.org (for resources for teaching and training in adolescent health).

## Practical points for communicating and working with adolescents

- See young people by themselves as well as with their parents. Do not exclude parents completely, but make it clear that the adolescent is the centre of the consultation. Do this routinely as a way of respecting their healthcare rights
- Be empathic, respectful, and non-judgmental, particularly when discussing behaviours such as substance misuse that may result in harm to the adolescent
- Assure confidentiality in all clinical settings
- Be yourself. Don't try to be cool or hip—young people want you to be their doctor, not their friend
- Try to communicate and explain concepts in a manner appropriate to their development. For young adolescents, use only "here and now" concrete examples and avoid abstract concepts ("if . . . then") discussions
- If appropriate, take a full adolescent psychosocial history (the HEADSS protocol is helpful for this—see next box)

## HEADSS protocol

*H—Home life including relationship with parents

E—Education or employment, including financial issues

A—Activities including sports (also particularly note friendships and social relationships, especially close friendships)

A—Affect (mood, particularly whether mood is responsive to situations)

D—Drug use, including cigarettes and alcohol as well as drugs

S—Sex (information on intimate relationships and sexual risk behaviours may be important in both acute and chronic illnesses in adolescents)

S—Suicide, depression, and self harm

S—Sleep

*Adapted from Goldenring et al. *Contemporary Pediatrics* 1998;Jul:75-80

# 2 Consent, competence, and confidentiality

Vic Larcher

Adolescence represents the final phase in the transition from the dependence of infancy to the autonomy of adulthood. It can be difficult for young people, parents, and health professionals alike, because of the nature and speed of change. Uncertainty over ethical and legal rights and responsibilities may lead professionals to refuse to see adolescents aged under 16 years on their own for fear of incurring parental wrath or even legal action. Disputes may arise in relation to an adolescent's competence to seek, consent to, or refuse medical treatment, and his or her right to confidentiality. In most cases these disputes can be resolved by discussion, compromise, and partnership, but in extreme circumstances the courts may be involved.

## Ethical and legal principles

All professionals have a duty to act in the best interests of their patients. Adults have the right to decide what their best interests are and to have their choices respected. Legally, adolescents' rights to make decisions for themselves depend on their ability to do so (called competence). Ethically, however, professionals have a duty to respect the rights of adolescents, irrespective of their ability to make decisions for themselves, provided that to respect these rights does not result in harm to the adolescent or to others (as laid down in the UN Convention on the Rights of the Child).

The legal principle underpinning provision of health care for children (under 18s) in the United Kingdom is that their best interests (welfare) are paramount. Legal duties are defined both by statute—for example, the Children Act 1989 and the UK Human Rights Act 1998—and by common law, which derives general principles from specific cases. UK law respects the rights of families to privacy, autonomy, and minimal outside intervention but acknowledges that parental rights decline during adolescence. In deciding best interests, courts apply the welfare checklist of the Children Act and consider relevant articles from the Human Rights Act.

## Consent for medical treatment

Obtaining consent for medical treatment respects the right of young people to self determination. To be legally valid, consent must be sufficiently informed and be freely given by a person who is competent to do so.

If young people lack the competence to make decisions, parents have the legal power to consent on their behalf. Matters are more complex when young people are competent but oppose their parents' wishes or refuse treatment.

## Competence

Many adolescents are competent in that they possess qualities associated with self determination—that is, cognitive ability, rationality, self identity, and ability to reason hypothetically. Many are able to consider how their actions affect others as well as themselves. In law an adolescent's competence is defined by their capacity to perform the task in question. Some tasks—such as owning pets and driving cars—are defined by age.

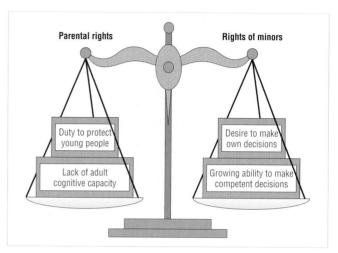

Balancing rights and responsibilities in adolescent care

---

**Welfare checklist of the Children Act**

- The ascertainable wishes and feelings of the young person concerned in the light of their age and understanding
- Physical, emotional, and educational needs
- Likely effect of change of circumstances
- Age, sex, cultural, religious, and ethnic background
- Harm or risk of harm
- Capability of parents or others to meet the young person's needs

---

**Relevant human rights (UK Human Rights Act 1998)**

*Article 2*—Right to life
*Article 3*—Prohibition of torture and inhuman and degrading treatment
*Article 5*—Right to liberty
*Article 8*—Right to respect for privacy and family life, home, and correspondence
*Article 9*—Freedom of thought, conscience, and religion
*Article 10*—Freedom of expression and right to information
*Article 12*—Right to marry and found a family
*Article 14*—Right not to be discriminated against on grounds of race, sex, etc, in the enjoyment of other convention rights

---

**Those allowed to give consent for treatment for young people**

- The young person if he or she either is over 16 years or is under 16 years and judged to be competent
- Parents, individuals, or local authority with parental responsibility
- A court

---

**Legal definition of competence**

"As a matter of law, the parental right to determine whether or not the minor child below the age of 16 will have medical treatment terminates if and when the child achieves sufficient understanding and intelligence to understand fully what is proposed" (Gillick v West Norfolk and Wisbech Area Health Authority [1985] 3 All ER 402HL)

The validity of a child's consent turns on personal capacity as judged by the opinion of a qualified medical practitioner attending him (Age of Legal Capacity (Scotland) Act 1991;S2(4).)

In health care, however, understanding, intelligence, and experience are important qualities. Over the age of 18 years competence is presumed. In England, Wales, and Northern Ireland adolescents aged 16-18 can consent to treatment but cannot necessarily refuse treatment intended to save their lives or prevent serious harm. Adolescents under 16 may legally consent if they satisfy certain criteria. This is easy for uncomplicated procedures such as venepuncture but is more problematic for complex, risky procedures such as open heart surgery. In Scotland competent children may consent to treatment irrespective of age; a person may make decisions on a young person's behalf only if the young person lacks the capacity to do so.

Competence is context dependent and may fluctuate. Pain, environment, and mental state may reduce competence, but experience of illness may increase it. In law, assessing competence is the doctor's responsibility, though other professionals with appropriate skills may be delegated to help. Refusal to cooperate with assessment should not lead to a presumption of incompetence. Some competent adolescents may wish to share decision making with trusted adults or let others decide for them. Assessment of competence must be done in situations that maximise competence—after giving adequate information in an appropriate environment..

## Information

Any competent adolescent can legally authorise medical procedures provided that they have the information that a reasonable person making a choice in similar circumstances would want.

The extent to which parents are involved needs sensitive handling. Adolescents may wish to ask intensely private questions —for example, on sexual matters—that exclude their parents.

Parents may wish to protect young people from painful and distressing facts—for example, about their own illnesses—but failure to disclose such information may cause more subsequent pain and suffering to the adolescent. Some families and cultures may not wish to involve young people in decision making. Adolescents not able or not wanting to make their own choices still have the right to information in a comprehensible form.

## Refusal

Refusal is especially problematic when the proposed treatment will prevent death or significant harm and the risk-benefit ratio is favourable—for example, an appendicectomy for acute appendicitis.

When the risk-benefits are more equivocal a wider consideration of best interests is necessary. Legal intervention may be necessary if disputes cannot be resolved by negotiation and mediation. Courts have overturned adolescents' refusal of psychiatric medication, blood transfusion in leukaemia, and heart lung transplantation.

## Confidentiality

Teenagers rate confidentiality as one of the most important aspects of medical care as it underpins future relationships with professionals and is based on mutual trust.

They wish to know that information given in confidence will not be divulged to others—for example, parents, school, and police—unless they specifically wish. They may test professional assurances of confidentiality. The right to confidentiality exists independently of the competence to consent to treatment.

---

**Criteria for testing competence**

The young person should be able to:
- Understand simple terms, nature, purpose, and necessity for proposed treatment
- Understand benefits/risks/alternatives and effect of non-treatment
- Believe the information applies to them
- Retain information long enough to make a choice
- Make a choice free from pressure

---

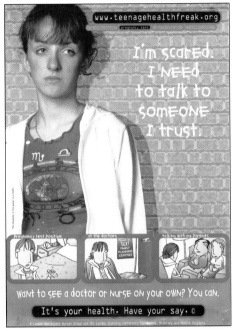

Adolescents have the right to receive information in a form and at a pace that they can assimilate and in an environment that respects their privacy and dignity and spares them embarrassment

---

**Coercion**
- Subtle forms of coercion on young people are common
- Failure to provide adequate time or facilities to receive and reflect on information may be coercive, even if unintentionally so
- Adolescents may feel that unquestioned agreement with authority figures such as doctors and parents is required
- Pressurising adolescents to make decisions when they feel neither happy nor confident to do so may be coercive

---

**Unlike for competent adults, an adolescent's right to refuse treatment depends on the circumstances**

---

**Refusal and forced treatments**
- Forcing adolescents to have treatments they do not want may produce long term psychological harms and lack of cooperation with future treatment
- Overriding an informed, sustained refusal by a competent adolescent is therefore only justified in extreme circumstances
- If adolescents refuse a minor or elective procedure, the procedure should be postponed
- The use of even reasonable physical restraint or force to provide treatment cannot be sanctioned unless the strongest possible justification exists
- Every attempt should be made to understand reasons for refusal and to remedy them
- Legal intervention should be used only when all other means of negotiation, including a careful explanation of the rights of all parties, have failed

## Situations in which confidentiality for adolescents is especially important

- Contraception
- Request by an unaccompanied young person for contraception or abortion
- Sexually transmitted infections
- Substance misuse, particularly illicit drugs
- Mental health issues

Objections to disclosure of information should mainly be honoured. Disclosure of information may be required by law or for the purpose of protecting the adolescent or others from risk of serious harm—namely, in the public interest. The adolescent should be told that information will be disclosed and the reasons for it.

Professionals may obtain practical guidance about disclosure from their own professional organisations or from their trust's legal services. Information leading to personal consequences—for example, informing agencies of a patient's epilepsy—should not be disclosed without consent unless public interest or legal obligation require it.

Particular problems may arise if an abused adolescent refuses permission to disclose information to social services or the police. Information about incompetent patients can be disclosed because it is in their best interests, and there is a statutory obligation to investigate abuse.

Similarly, attempts should be made to persuade competent adolescents to permit disclosure. In the face of sustained refusal, disclosure must be justified by a belief that there is a serious risk of harm to the adolescent or to others. Adolescents should be informed of the intention to disclose unless to do so would place them at further risk of harm.

Matters relating to sexual health—such as contraception, treatment of sexually transmitted diseases, and termination of pregnancy—are also problematic in that issues of competence and confidentiality may coexist. Legal guidance in handling such situations does exist and is equally applicable to issues other than contraception. Adverse consequences may follow if an adolescent's concern about confidentiality leads them to specialist clinics that do not have access to their full health records.

## Communicating with adolescents about treatment options and establishing competence

### General principles

- Treat adolescents as you would competent adults unless you have reason to doubt their competence
- Guarantee confidentiality unless there are specific reasons to break it
- Make every effort to involve their family (Fraser guidelines)
- Use open ended questions that prompt discussion
- Use colloquialisms but not jargon
- Be non-judgmental—make no presumptions about the young person's views or abilities
- Aim to increase their competence
- Encourage young people to express their own views
- Challenge expectations that adults hold decision making power

### Specific issues

- Ascertain what the young person knows about their illness or problem and its treatment
- Ascertain their personal experience of illness
- Ascertain their previous experience of decision making for their condition or issue—for example, whether they have been previously involved with parents' decision making

## Practical methods to help ensure confidentiality

### Have a surgery or clinic policy on confidentiality

- Ensure all staff know the policy and agree to interact with adolescents confidentially
- Put up posters for staff areas about the professional duty of confidentiality and details about legal and ethical issues
- Ensure staff are aware that young people are legally allowed to examine their own health records (if competent to do so and disclosure is unlikely to cause significant harm)
- Ensure confidentiality when appointments are booked and during telephone calls

### Make sure adolescents are aware of confidentiality policies

Ensure that adolescents are aware of confidentiality policies and practices of the surgery or clinic—for example, through waiting room posters

### Consider the implications of confidentiality

Consider the implications for confidentiality of non-therapeutic activities that require sharing of anonymised data, which may be disclosed without consent but with the knowledge of the adolescent concerned—such as audit, research, teaching, service planning

## Situations in which confidentiality should not be kept when dealing with young people

### With a competent young person

- Disclosure of history of or current sexual abuse
- Disclosure of current or recent suicidal thoughts or significant self-harming behaviour
- Disclosure of homicidal intent

### With an incompetent young person

- Any situation in which there is a significant risk of harm to the adolescent or to others

## Fraser guidelines* on young people's competence to consent to contraceptive advice or treatment

A young person is competent to consent to contraceptive advice or treatment if:

- The young person understands the doctor's advice
- The doctor cannot persuade the young person to inform his or her parents or allow the doctor to inform the parents that he or she is seeking contraceptive advice
- The young person is very likely to begin or continue having sexual intercourse with or without contraceptive treatment
- The young person's physical or mental health or both are likely to deteriorate if he or she does not receive contraceptive advice or treatment
- The young person's best interests require the doctor to give contraceptive advice or treatment, or both, without parent consent

*Gillick v West Norfolk and Wisbech Area Health Authority [1985] 3 All ER 402HL

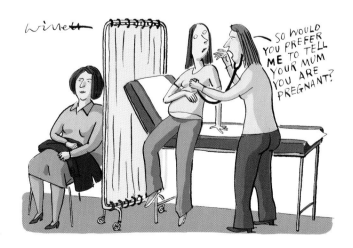

# Conclusions

Issues of consent and confidentiality are central in many clinical interactions with adolescents. Services that are not considered confidential are considerably less likely to be used by young people. Those who work with young people must have a clear understanding of consent and confidentiality and also ensure that the services they work in have policies and practices that increase confidentiality and competence among teenage patients.

**"Good parenting involves giving minors as much rope as they can handle without an unacceptable risk that they will hang themselves" Lord Donaldson in Re W [1992] 4 All ER 627-633**

**Much the same can be said for adolescent medicine**

The poster is published with permission of London Adolescent Network Group.

---

**Further reading and resources**

- British Medical Association. *Consent, rights and choices in health care for children and young people.* London: BMJ Books, 2001.
- Royal College of Paediatrics and Child Health. *Responsibilities of doctors in child protection cases with regard to confidentiality.* London: RCPCH, 2004.
- General Medical Council. *Confidentiality: protecting and providing information.* London: GMC, 2000.
- Alderson P, Montgomery J. Health care choices: making decisions with children. London: Institute for Public Policy Research, 1996.
- Department of Health. *Best practice guidance for doctors and other health professionals on the provision of advice and treatment to young people under 16 on contraception, sexual, and reproductive health.* London: DoH, 2004. (Gateway reference No 3382.)
- "Confidentiality Toolkit" (a pack designed to help general practice teams review and develop their policy on confidentiality), available free from the Royal College of General Practitioners (tel 020 7581 3232; email sales@rcgp.org.uk).

# 3   Epidemiology of health and illness

Russell Viner, Robert Booy

Adolescents constitute a large percentage of the population, have a distinct pattern of health and illness, and are one subset of the population that has experienced little or least improvement in overall health status over the past 40 years.

## The youth demographic

In most developed countries young people aged between 10 and 20 years account for 13-15% of the population. The World Health Organization classifies young people as 10-24 year olds, with adolescence (10-19 years) and youth (15-24 years) overlapping within that age range. There were 7.6 million adolescents aged 10-19 years in the United Kingdom in mid-2000, making up 12.7% of the population. Projections suggest that the numbers of adolescents will grow by 8.5% between 1998 and 2011.

Health problems among adolescents seem to be increasing. This partly reflects a rise in the proportions of black and other ethnic minority groups in the adolescent population. Ethnic diversity is greater in young people than in the general UK population, and minority ethnicity is linked to poor health outcomes in adolescence, such as suicide, teenage pregnancy, sexually transmitted infections, and mental disorders; the most plausible link is through socioeconomic disadvantage.

## Patterns of disease and health risk

Disease and health behaviours in adolescents have patterns that are distinct from those of children or adults. In particular, adolescent mortality and morbidity rates show worrying trends in national priority areas such as mental health—for example, male suicide, sexual health (teenage pregnancy and sexually transmitted infections), and cardiovascular risk (obesity and type 2 diabetes).

## Mortality

The considerable recent improvements seen in mortality in 1-4 year olds have not been matched in adolescents, and death rates among 15-19 year olds are now higher than in the 1-4 year age group. This is due to the rise of "social" causes of mortality, including road traffic injuries, other injuries, and suicide, which have replaced communicable diseases as the most common causes of death in adolescents.

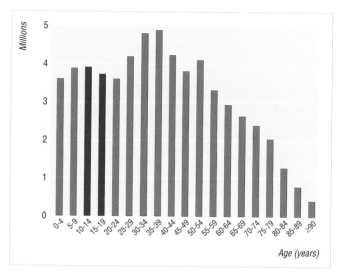

UK population by age, mid-2000

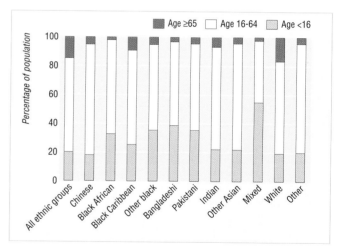

Age distribution of ethnic groups in United Kingdom, 2001-2

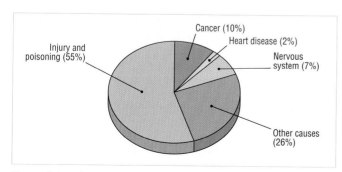

Causes of death in 15-19 year olds in United Kingdom, 1997

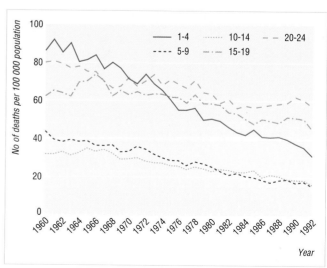

Mortality by age group in United Kingdom, 1960-92

9

**Road traffic injuries**

Road traffic injuries are the leading cause of death in adolescence (with road traffic accidents causing 27% of deaths in 15-24 year olds), particularly in young men, with motor vehicle collisions the main contributor. This contrasts strongly with mortality for all adults, in whom traffic injuries account for 1-2% of deaths. Far from being random events, road traffic injuries in young people are strongly associated with risk factors such as alcohol, depression, social disruption, and stress. Transport patterns are an important determinant of health in adolescence, and transport is one area where health promotion strategies could greatly reduce mortality in this age group.

**Suicide**

Suicide by young males has become one of the most worrying public health issues for developed countries in the past three decades. In the United Kingdom, the suicide rate for older male teenagers almost doubled between 1970 and 1988 and remained high through to the late 1990s. This has occurred alongside a doubling in the rate of deaths from undetermined causes for this group during the same period, suggesting that many suicides may still be unreported. Comparable data from other developed countries show similar trends.

# Drugs and alcohol

Regular alcohol drinking (defined as once a week or more) in the United Kingdom rises from 3% of 11 year olds to 38% of 15 year olds, with boys and girls nearly equal until age 15.

Like smoking and drinking, the prevalence of drug misuse in adolescence increases sharply with age. In 1998, only 1% of 11 year olds in England had ever tried drugs, compared with 31% of 15 year olds.

The likelihood of having ever used drugs is strongly related to smoking and drinking experience. Few adolescents who have never smoked or drunk try drugs, but up to three quarters of regular smokers who drink at least once a week have tried drugs. Similar risk and protective factors to those for smoking operate for substance use, with depression a particular risk factor.

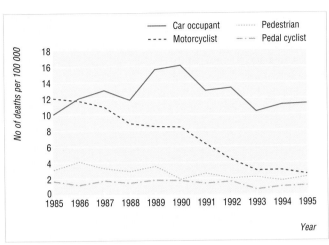

Male death rates related to road traffic injuries among teenagers aged 15-19 years in England and Wales, 1985-95. Adapted from DiGiuseppi et al (*BMJ* 1998;316;904-5)

> **Alcohol misuse disorders in adolescence are not benign conditions; they often continue into adulthood and are associated with later substance misuse, depression, and antisocial behaviours**

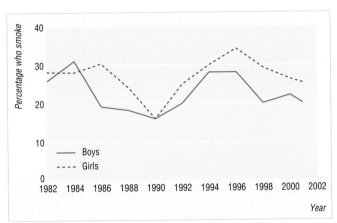

Prevalence of cigarette smoking among 15-16 year olds in England, 1982-2001. Adapted from Coleman and Schofield (see Further Reading box)

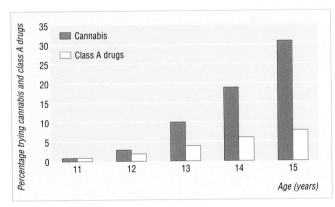

Proportions of 11-15 year olds in England who have ever tried cannabis or class A drugs (heroin, methadone, cocaine, ecstasy, LSD, injected amphetamines), by age, 2001. Adapted from Coleman and Schofield (see Further Reading box)

# Teenage pregnancy and sexual health

Teenage pregnancy rates in the United Kingdom are among the highest in western Europe. Teenage mothers have poorer antenatal health, have children with poorer health, have poorer health themselves, and have poorer educational and financial outcomes later in life. Key risk factors for teenage pregnancy include poverty, living in a city, poor parental supervision, low

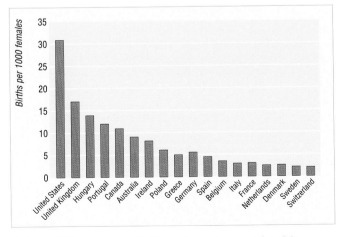

Births per 1000 women aged 15-17 years in member countries of the Organisation for Economic Co-operation and Development, 1998. Adapted from Coleman and Schofield (see Further Reading box)

educational expectations, and lack of access to services; many of these factors probably relate to social disadvantage.

Rates of sexually transmitted infection increased greatly among teenagers in the late 1990s. Between 1993 and 1999 the overall rate of diagnoses of uncomplicated chlamydia among 16-19 year olds presenting to genitourinary medicine clinics more than doubled, from 340 to 791 per 100 000 population in females and from 90 to 216 per 100 000 population in males. These figures undoubtedly underestimate the rate of chlamydia in the community and indicate the need for screening young people for sexually transmitted infections.

## Mental health

Mental health problems during adolescence include the emergence of new mental health issues such as depression, early onset "adult" disorders such as schizophrenia, and the continuation of childhood problems such as attention-deficit/hyperactivity disorder and conduct disorder. The recent UK national mental health survey found that among 11-15 year olds, serious mental health problems are found in 13% of boys and 19% of girls, although if more minor problems are included, about a fifth of young people develop mental health problems during adolescence.

Eating disorders are now the third most common chronic condition of adolescence in girls, in whom it is nine times more common than in boys. Estimates of the prevalence of eating disorders are difficult because of subclinical or hidden problems, but it is estimated that among female adolescents about 0.5% have anorexia nervosa, 1% have bulimia nervosa, and 3% to 5% have subclinical syndromes.

## Obesity

Obesity now overshadows all other chronic illnesses in adolescents. Recent estimates based on the new definitions from the International Obesity TaskForce suggest that about 23% of UK 10-15 years olds are overweight and a further 6% are obese. At the root of these high levels of overweight and obesity is a population shift towards eating more calorie dense "fast foods," spending more time in sedentary activity such as playing computer games and watching television, and doing less physical activity. During the past 15 years in the United Kingdom, the average annual distance cycled by teenagers has fallen by 31% and the average annual distance walked has fallen by 24%; car travel during this period has increased by 35%.

## Chronic illness

The burden of chronic illness in adolescence is increasing in all developed countries as larger numbers of chronically ill children survive into their teens and 20s.

The most common chronic illnesses are respiratory conditions, and cohort studies in the United Kingdom show that the prevalence of wheezing at age 16 years rose by 70% between 1974 and 1986, with further rises in the 1990s. Other illnesses with substantial rises in incidence include type 1 diabetes (with an annual Europe-wide increase of 2.4% for 10-14 year olds during the past 10 years) and type 2 diabetes, particularly in ethnic minority populations. The particular dangers of the transition from paediatric to adult services is well illustrated by reports of totally inappropriate treatment of patients with congenital heart defects by cardiologists who work with adults with acquired heart disorders. Transition programmes, however, improve health outcomes and patients' quality of life.

**Sexually transmitted infections often occur in adolescents who engage in other risk behaviours (including substance misuse), have psychological disorders, and experience violence (or are violent themselves). Reporting rates of both gonorrhoea and syphilis have shown similar rises to chlamydia**

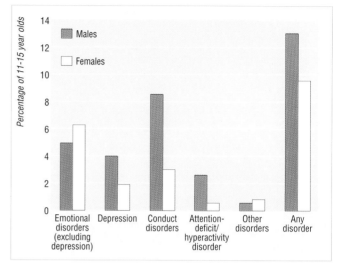

Prevalence of mental disorders in 11-15 year olds in United Kingdom, 1999

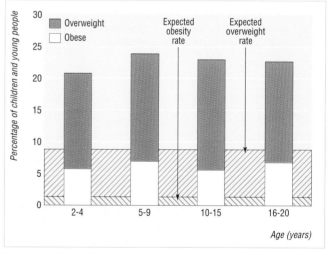

Prevalence of overweight and obesity (according to definitions of the International Obesity TaskForce) in English children and adolescents (health study for England, 1999). Expected rates (R Viner, unpublished data) are based on the task force definitions

**The prevalence of cystic fibrosis among people aged over 15 years in the United Kingdom more than doubled between 1977 and 1985, and currently over 85% of children with chronic illness survive to adulthood**

# Conclusions

Adolescence is generally a healthy period of life compared with early childhood and old age. However, the recent improvements in mortality seen in young children have not been matched in teenagers, and adolescent morbidity shows worrying trends in key areas such as mental health, sexual health, and cardiovascular risk. As behaviours that both increase and protect against poor health outcomes in later life are laid down in adolescence, increased public health, policy, and clinical focus on the health of young people will have important benefits for the long term health of the population.

---

### Further reading and resources

- Coleman J, Schofield J. *Key data on adolescence.* Trust for the Study of Adolescence, Brighton, 2003.
- Viner RM. Adolescent medicine. In: Warrell DA, Cox TM, Firth JD, Benz Jr EJ, eds. *Oxford textbook of medicine.* 4th ed. Oxford: Oxford University Press, 2003.
- Neinstein LS. *Adolescent health care: a practical guide.* Baltimore: Williams & Wilkins, 2002.
- www.euteach.com (for resources for teaching epidemiology in adolescent health)
- www.statistics.gov.uk (for data on young people in the United Kingdom)
- www.relachs.org (Research with East London Adolescents: Community Health Survey is a school based epidemiological study of adolescents in east London that provides insights into aspects of health and wellbeing of inner urban British adolescents)

---

**Health problems in adolescence, and adolescent behavioural and health problems that may lead to major health problems in later life\***

*Problems affecting young people disproportionately*—Accidental injury, intentional injury, substance misuse, teenage pregnancy, sexually transmitted infections, mental illness, suicide, depression, eating disorders, anxiety, attention-deficit/hyperactivity disorder, psychosis

*Problems persisting from childhood*—Chronic illness (such as asthma, diabetes, epilepsy, metabolic diseases, congenital heart disease), acute childhood illness (such as cancer and meningitis), conduct and behavioural disorders

*Behavioural and health problems leading to health problems later*—Obesity, physical inactivity, and poor diet; mental illness; substance misuse; sexually risky behaviour

\*Adapted from: Patton GC. *The scope for youth health development.* Melbourne, Australia: University of Melbourne, 1999

---

All the graphs are adapted from data on the website of the Office for National Statistics (www.statistics.gov.uk), except where stated otherwise.

# 4  Adolescents in primary care

Ann McPherson

The specific health needs of young people are often neglected by primary care as it is believed that adolescents are on the whole a healthy group who rarely present to their general practitioner (GP). "Out of sight" has been "out of mind," especially given the ever increasing pressures on primary care from other client groups.

The new GP contract in England and Wales has done nothing to mitigate this. Change is needed, however, as teenagers (a) have many health concerns, though they do not always tell their GP about them, and (b) do visit their GPs, on average two to three times a year (with about 70% of all teenagers visiting their GP in any one year). These visits provide opportunities to deal with their health concerns.

Surveys have shown that adolescents are usually happy to discuss health issues with their GP, but 40% say that they find it difficult to see their GP. Over 60% said that they would not know how to register with a GP when they left home, and 71% did not know how to register as a temporary resident. Young people identify confidentiality and access as the most important aspects of primary care for them.

A survey of all general practices in Oxfordshire showed that only about 30% of practices had tackled the issue of confidentiality and "user friendly" services for adolescents. These are the issues perceived by teenagers as the greatest barriers to accessing primary care.

---

**Barriers to primary care perceived by adolescents**
- Concerns about confidentiality
- Geographical barriers (such as difficult to get to by public transport)
- Lack of information about services
- Appointments and opening times unsuitable for young people
- Parental consent not obtainable
- Unfriendly environment and staff
- Language barriers (staff use jargon or overly "adult" language)

---

## Communication with young people

Effective communication is an essential part of any clinical interaction. Yet adolescents and doctors in primary care often feel that communication between these two groups is often highly problematic. Special skills are needed for effective clinical communication with adolescents—skills that require an understanding of cognitive and social development in adolescence and an ability to understand that the social contexts of health behaviours in adolescents can be very different from the contexts for children and adults.

One of the reasons that health professionals find communication with young people difficult is that this is the only time in clinical practice that they are not dealing direct with adults. When seeing adult patients, health workers communicate with other adults, who share largely similar social values and norms about health, even taking account of cultural differences. When seeing children, they negotiate treatment decisions with the parents, with children's participation being obtained by explanation and parental authority. In contrast, in consultations with adolescents, health professionals are faced with the challenge of communicating with a personality undergoing rapid psychological and social changes who may

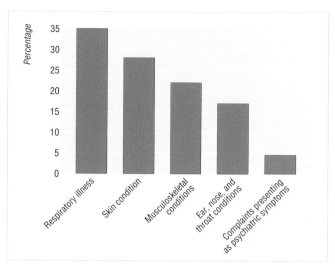

Reasons that teenagers visit their general practitioner. Data from Churchill et al. *Br J Gen Pract* 2000;50:953-7

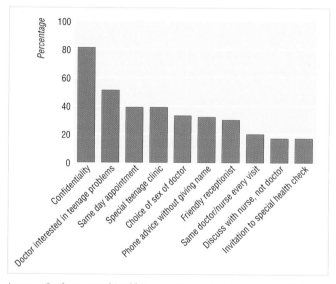

Aspects of primary care identified as most important to young people. Data from Donovan C et al. *Br J Gen Pract* 1997;47:715-8

---

**Communicating with young people**
- Be clear that you will respect their privacy and confidentiality
- See young people by themselves (time consuming and perhaps difficult to arrange but essential for providing enough confidential space for discussion)
- Be patient (teenagers may need further consultations before they trust you enough)
- Ask open ended questions to draw out information
- Listen more than you talk
- Use terms the adolescent will understand
- Do not be judgmental about their values and opinions unless these place them at clear risk

**Particular issues for younger teenagers**
- Use concrete language and expect concrete questions and answers
- As teenagers get older and their developmental capacities change, you may need to repeat information provided earlier
- Remember that teenagers often feel a conflict between a desire to be independent and a need to remain dependent on their parents

---

not share an adult's understanding of society or adult cognitive abilities to decide between treatments in the light of future risks to health.

Randomised controlled trials show, however, that training can improve GPs' communication skills and interactions with young people (Sanci et al, see "Further reading" box). But do not be tempted to seem too "hip" or "cool" in interactions with teenagers. Young people want you to be their doctor, not their friend.

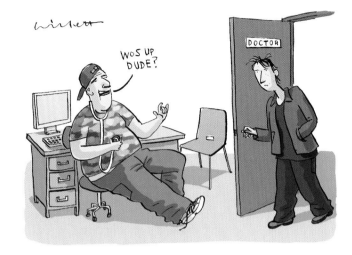

# Improving primary care services

The following ideas show how primary care services for adolescents can be improved. Many of the suggestions can be implemented without a lot of time and resources.

## Improve friendliness of the practice

Young people rate friendliness as a high priority for a general practice, so organise a meeting for all practice staff (including the secretaries and receptionists) to look at ways of making the practice more friendly for teenagers. Use role play to identify the issues that might arise for the young person in the practice. Audit what your practice currently provides for young people.

## Identify needs of teenage patients

Doing a "needs assessment" of your practice is one of the first steps towards making a practice adolescent friendly. It is relatively easy to work out your practice's adolescent profile using the practice's age and sex register and the knowledge of individual team members.

## Train staff appropriately

All practice staff need to be trained about their interaction with teenagers. In specific areas, such as contraception, staff need to be sensitive to young people's embarrassment—if staff respond inappropriately, teenagers may not return to the practice.

Advertise clearly in the waiting room, for example, that emergency contraception is available, and make sure that the receptionists do not ask embarrassing questions about emergency appointments. If a doctor is unwilling to give emergency contraception, make sure that the young person will be directed towards alternative sources of help without being made to feel guilty.

## Inform about practice services

Posters about the services that the practice provides for young people are useful so that when they attend for one problem they know that they can get advice on other issues—for example, contraception, depression, and drugs.

Consider also compiling a "practice information" booklet for teenagers. It's also a good idea to write a "birthday letter" to all young people when they become 16 (or earlier), explaining about the practice and pointing out that they may register with their choice of GP when they become 16 and get contraceptive services from any GP willing to offer the service.

## Prioritise confidentiality

Adolescents are used to the fact that much of what they say about themselves and the way they behave is not treated as confidential by their family, friends, peers, and teachers.

Contact with the primary healthcare team may be the first time that the concept of confidentiality will be raised. It is essential that the practice conveys a positive message about confidentiality.

---

**Is your practice "user friendly" for young people?**

- Are there posters and leaflets in the waiting room (or toilets) directed at young people?
- Are the leaflets user friendly—glossy, lots of pictures, suitable language?
- Do you provide appropriate information on counselling services (such as Childline) or drug services?

---

**Doing a needs assessment**

- Determine the total number of young people aged 10-18 in the practice (with age bands, by sex)
- Determine the percentage of young people seen in the past year
- Determine the number seen for sensitive issues such as contraceptive advice
- Identify the practice staff who see young people
- Identify the practice staff with special skills or training in working with young people
- Ask your staff about areas of working with young people that they would like more training in
- Ask young people in your practice what improvements they want

---

**It is worth telling young people and their parents how they can a register as a temporary patient**

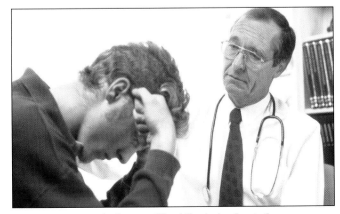

Reassure young people about confidentiality during face to face consultations

- Use posters such "Here to listen not to tell" (available from Brook, a UK charity providing free and confidential sexual health advice and services for young people aged under 25; www.brook.org.uk)
- Consider displaying the booklet *Private and Confidential— Talking to Doctors* (available from Brook)
- Every member of the practice needs to understand the confidentiality "code of practice" and be familiar with the "confidentiality toolkit" (available from the Royal College of General Practitioners, tel 020 7581 3232; sales@rcgp.org.uk).

### Organise a young persons clinic

These are successful in some practices and not in others, and how well they work usually depends on, for example, the personality of the person running them, the characteristics of the local teenage population, and whether other local general practices join in.

### Involve parents

During the teenage years parents still continue to be the main providers, carers, and sources of health information to teenagers. This contribution by parents needs to be supported and respected. Provide information for parents about the practice's facilities for teenagers and other resources (on, for example, depression, drugs, and eating disorders). Make sure that parents know how to tell their teenagers about contraception (including emergency contraception). Discuss with young people the advantages of involving their parents in sexually related decisions.

### Support for pregnant teenagers

If a teenager gets pregnant, make sure that they are given support and help in coming to a decision on whether to continue with the pregnancy or have a termination—without indulging in moral attitudes.

If they want to continue with the pregnancy try to get them to involve their parents and put them in contact with supporting agencies, including the health visitor. If they decide to have a termination arrange for a rapid referral. If you are against a termination, ensure that the young person is not made to feel guilty and arrange for them to see another doctor immediately.

### Advise young men, too

It is important to remember young men as well as women, so let them know they are also welcome at your practice. In advertising contraceptive services, direct the information at both boys and girls.

Consider providing free condoms and advising about emergency contraception and sexually transmitted infections. Try putting up posters in your waiting room that are aimed directly at young men. Run clinics specifically for young men, although these may work best in a community centre rather than in your clinic.

The photograph of a young person with his doctor is published with permission from CC Studio/SPL; and the photograph of the pregnant girl is with permission from Clare Marsh/John Birdsall Library.

---

**It is a good idea to advertise to adolescents what sources of help are available to them locally, outside the practice services. They need to know about, for example, young people's clinics (including Brook), family planning clinics, other general practices, accident and emergency departments, and condom machines in lavatories**

---

### Issues in setting up a young persons clinic

- It takes time not only for teenagers to find out about them but also to have confidence in them
- The timing needs to be convenient for teenagers—that is, immediately after school
- Consider running the clinic with the school nurse in the school setting or in other less medical community settings
- Make the environment teenage friendly—ask teenagers how this can be done

---

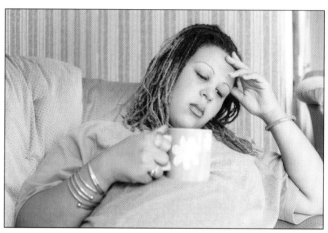

Support the teenager, whatever decision she makes about her pregnancy

---

### Further reading and resources

- McPherson A, Macfarlane A, Allen J. What do young people want from their GP? *Br J Gen Pract* 1996;46:627.
- Kari J, Donovan C, Li J, Taylor B. Adolescents' attitudes to general practice in north London. *Br J Gen Pract* 1997;47:109-10.
- Gregg R, Freeth D, Blackie C. Teenage health and the practice nurse: choice and opportunity for both? *Br J Gen Pract* 1998;48:909-10.
- Jacobson L, Mellanby A, Donovan C, Taylor B, Tripp J, members of the Adolescent Working Party, Royal College of General Practitioners. Teenagers' views on general practice consultations and other medical advice. *Fam Pract* 2000;17:156-8.
- Sanci L, Coffey C, Veit F, Carr-Gregg M, Patton G, Day N, Bowes G. Evaluation of an educational intervention for general practitioners in adolescent health care: randomised controlled trial. *BMJ* 2000;320:224-2.
- *Clueless* and *Trust*—Training videos (10 minutes long) about teenagers and primary healthcare services for use in general practice to prompt discussion on how to improve primary healthcare services for young people. Available from the Royal College of General Practitioners (tel 020 7581 3232; sales@rcgp.org.uk), price £7 each.

# 5 Chronic illness and disability

Michele Yeo, Susan Sawyer

Young people with chronic conditions often face more difficulties negotiating the tasks of adolescence than their healthy peers. National, population based studies from Western countries show that 20-30% of teenagers have a chronic illness, defined as one that lasts longer than six months. However, 10-13% of teenagers report having a chronic condition that substantially limits their daily life or requires extended periods of care and supervision.

The burden of chronic conditions in adolescence is increasing as larger numbers of chronically ill children survive beyond the age of 10. Over 85% of children with congenital or chronic conditions now survive into adolescence, and conditions once seen only in young children are now seen beyond childhood and adolescence. In addition, the prevalence of certain chronic illnesses in adolescence, such as diabetes (types 1 and 2) and asthma, has increased, as has survival from cancer.

## Impact of chronic conditions on adolescence

Chronic conditions in adolescence can affect physical, cognitive, social, and emotional spheres of development for adolescents, with repercussions for siblings and parents too.

### Physical effects

Common sequelae of chronic illness and its treatment include short stature and pubertal delay. Undernutrition is common in many chronic conditions, and obesity can result from conditions that limit physical activity. Visible signs of illness or its treatment mark young people out as different at a time when such differences are important to young people and their peers. Body image issues related to height, weight, pubertal stage, and scarring can contribute to reduced self esteem and negative self image, problems that may persist into adult life.

### Emotional and mental health

Many young people cope well with the emotional aspects of having a chronic illness. Chronically ill young people are more likely, however, to have a lower level of emotional wellbeing than their healthy peers. Young people often report a sense of alienation from their peers and frustration with the requirements of managing their condition and negotiating the healthcare system.

Young people with chronic illness do not have an increased rate of mental illness, as is the case in adults with chronic illness. However, because those with chronic illness experience many sources of stress, health professionals must be alert for depression, anxiety, and adjustment disorders both in young people and in their families. Behavioural problems and declining school performance can be specific markers of underlying psychological distress in adolescence.

### Social, educational, and vocational aspects

Effects of chronic illness on cognition and learning can be subtle, often manifesting as poor performance at school—largely the result of repeated absence because of poor health or

## Prevalence (per 1000 adolescents aged 12-18 years) of certain chronic conditions in mid-adolescence

|  | Prevalence |
| --- | --- |
| Musculoskeletal conditions: | 41 |
| Cerebral palsy | 15 |
| Skin conditions | 32 |
| Serious mental health problems: | 120* |
| Anorexia or bulimia nervosa | 15 |
| Attention-deficit/hyperactivity disorder | 100* |
| Diabetes: | |
| Type 1 | 2 |
| Type 2 | 1-2 |
| Respiratory conditions: | 150* |
| Asthma | 100* |
| Cystic fibrosis | 0.1 |
| Epilepsy | 4 |
| Ear or hearing problems | 18 |

*Uncertain value owing to differences in disease definitions

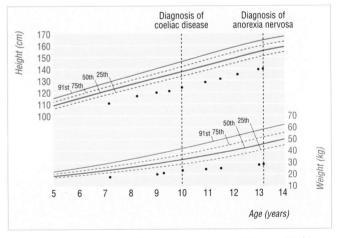

Growth chart (with 25th, 50th, 75th, and 91st centiles) of 13 year old girl with coeliac disease and anorexia nervosa. Coeliac disease was diagnosed at age 10 during investigation for short stature. She later presented, at age 13, with mother's concerns about restriction of food

## Features of depression in adolescence

- Low mood and tearfulness
- Moodiness and emotional outbursts
- Boredom
- Withdrawal and isolation
- Feelings of hopelessness and helplessness
- Changes in appetite and eating behaviour
- Disturbed sleep (such as greatly increased sleep and early or frequent waking)
- Fatigue
- Highly impulsive behaviour, risk taking behaviour (such as alcohol misuse, crime)
- Psychosomatic symptoms
- Poor school performance
- Preoccupation with death (in the media, clothing, art, music)
- Suicidal ideation
- Decrease in treatment adherence or in interest in managing their health

admission to hospital. Young people with chronic illness are at greater risk of social isolation owing to school absenteeism and lack of participation in recreational and sporting activities. Together with educational disadvantage, this means that young people with chronic conditions may find great difficulty getting jobs and achieving financial independence as adults.

Health professionals must help to improve young people's transition from education to the workforce. They can do this in several ways. They should encourage development of vocational capacity in the same way as for healthy young people: encouraging employment in part time jobs and working for parents; identifying suitable work experience placements; and identifying strengths and abilities rather than disabilities. They should start these strategies in early adolescence. Health professionals should also continually reassess the young person's vocational readiness in terms of educational achievement, communication skills, self esteem, expectations, and work experience.

## Impact of chronic conditions on families

Normal parenting issues in adolescence are amplified by chronic conditions. Chronic illness can hinder the young person's progression towards autonomy, keeping them dependent on their parents just when they are needing more independence. Additional time is needed to care for the young person, which generally carries a financial burden. It is not uncommon for parents to experience guilt, frustration, anxiety, and depression. Specific support services can be useful, and family therapy may be helpful. Siblings are also at greater risk of adjustment difficulties as they often miss out on parental time and attention and may be excluded from family discussions.

## Treatment: adherence and concordance

Health professionals aim to achieve the best treatment of the condition, often resulting in a focus on future benefit from current behaviour. In contrast, young people are influenced by the "here and now" and are more interested in achieving the goals of adolescence than improving their health. This can lead to conflicting priorities between the young person and his or her health professionals (and parents).

Health professionals can make the treatment goals more relevant for the young person by identifying how the illness affects them in terms of their appearance, ability to socialise well, or recreational opportunities. The task for health professionals is to work with the young person to develop concrete short term goals (weeks to months), such as focusing on good enough health to attend the school camp in four to six weeks' time. Active participation in negotiation of treatment plans helps young people to take back some ownership and control of the disease from the parents. Adolescents should have an understanding of their illness, especially the rationale for treatment and treatment options. Information must be provided at a level that is developmentally and cognitively appropriate.

Families can be a major source of support around adherence to treatment. Young people who come from cohesive families with open communication channels and lower levels of stress adhere better to treatment regimens and have better long term health outcomes. Trusted peers may also be involved as positive sources of support.

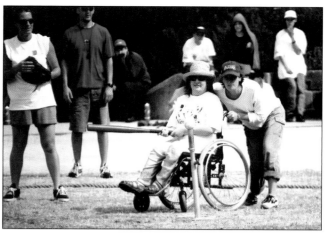

Young people with a chronic condition who can take part in recreational and sporting activities with their peers may be less likely to be socially isolated

---

**Effect of adolescence on chronic illness**

- The developmental changes of adolescence will reciprocally affect chronic illness and its management
- Smoking can exacerbate health outcomes in young people with asthma, cystic fibrosis, and diabetes
- Alcohol and dance parties can complicate diabetes care
- Exhaustion from late night parties can lead to unstable epilepsy
- For physiological reasons certain diseases can become more unstable during adolescence (the hormonal changes of the pubertal growth spurt decrease insulin sensitivity and make diabetes more difficult to control; lung function often deteriorates during adolescence in those with cystic fibrosis, especially girls)

---

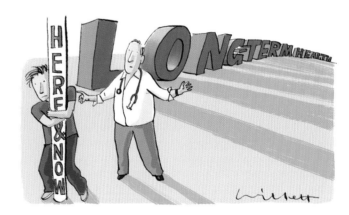

---

**Improving treatment adherence in adolescents**

- See the young person alone and discuss confidentiality
- Use a non-judgmental approach and ask open ended questions
- When asking about medication use, indicate to the young person that poor adherence to treatment is normal behaviour
- Explore what the young person knows about health and correct any misunderstandings
- Educate the young person about his or her illness and treatment
- Negotiate short term treatment goals
- Use the simplest regimen
- Tailor the regimen to the young person's daily routines
- Identify and discuss any potential barriers to adherence
- Explain the treatment regimen and repeat the instructions
- Give written instructions
- Avoid jargon in oral and written instructions
- Suggest reminders—for example, stickers on the bathroom mirror, medication calendar
- Enlist the support of parents, significant adults, trusted peers
- Review treatment and monitor adherence frequently—give useful feedback

Efforts to improve adherence should be routine in all consultations with young people. After hearing the parental perspective, seeing the young person alone for part of the consultation is important. A non-judgmental approach that accepts that poor adherence is relatively normal behaviour encourages the young person to be more honest when reporting less than ideal behaviour (for example, "Most people I see your age have difficulty taking medication regularly. Tell me, how are things going with you? Are you more likely to forget your morning or evening medication?"). Specifically inquire about adherence to each aspect of their healthcare regimen.

## Primary care

The normal primary healthcare needs of those with chronic illness are often neglected. The general practitioner is a key link with schools and community agencies. The general practitioner's knowledge of the family means they can offer support to parents and siblings alike. Health promotion should not be forgotten, whether it relates to nutrition, sexual health, or health risk behaviours such as smoking and drinking.

## Transition to adult services

Young people who need ongoing specialist care beyond adolescence must transfer to adult services. How the transfer takes place can depend on the availability of local services and the extent of specialist involvement. The care can be transferred, for example, from a specialist paediatric service either direct to an adult service or via an adolescent or young adult service (which may be located within either the paediatric or the adult service). The general practitioner can provide an important source of continuity during the change between specialty practitioners (including, for example, liaison with occupational therapists and physiotherapists), although this can be difficult in some highly specialised chronic illnesses.

Young people and their parents need information about the transition process and time to prepare. Parental anxieties that the adult team will not be able to cater for their teenager's healthcare needs are a common barrier to successful transition. Good communication between the paediatric and adult healthcare teams is important for smooth transition.

Transfer should take place when young people are developmentally ready and have the necessary set of skills to cope well in adult services, rather than at a fixed age. Primary care can play its part in promoting a smooth transition by encouraging independence in consultations with young people—for example, by seeing young people by themselves as well as with their parents—and beginning this process in early adolescence.

The photograph of the disabled girl taking part in sport was supplied by the authors.

**Importance of routine in adherence**

- A routine—or the lack of one—can affect adherence in young people, who often have a routine for one dose or treatment but not for another
- An example of an evening routine resulting in good adherence may include cleaning their teeth, setting their alarm clock, and then taking their medication
- The lack of morning routines around medication is common—often related to rushing before school
- Tailor their treatment regimens to make them as simple as possible
- Regular review provides an opportunity to remind the young person of how they can better monitor their health or adhere to their medication regimen, even in a small way

---

**The transfer of an adolescent from child centred to adult oriented healthcare systems is an important transition and one that is more complex than the simple transfer of the medical record from one institution or doctor to another**

---

**Key points for transition from paediatric services to adult services**

- Transition preparation is an essential component of high quality health care in adolescence
- Every paediatric general and specialty clinic should have a transition policy; more formal transition programmes are needed if large numbers of young people are being transferred to adult care
- Young people should not be transferred to adult services until they have the skills to function in an adult service and have finished growth and puberty
- Preparation for transition should start early—well before entering adolescence
- Personalised transition plans are needed for each young person
- An identified person (ideally a nurse specialist) in the paediatric and adult teams must be responsible for transition arrangements
- Management links must be developed between the two services
- Transition arrangements should be evaluated

---

**Adolescents with chronic illness have the same developmental needs as their healthy peers. Attention must be paid to developmental outcomes if good health outcomes are to be achieved**

---

**Further reading and resources**

- Neinstein LS. *Adolescent health care: a practical guide.* Baltimore, MD: Williams & Wilkins, 2002.
- Suris JC, Michaud PA, Viner R. The adolescent with a chronic condition: parts 1 and 2. *Arch Dis Child* 2004;89:938-49.
- www.connexions.gov.uk (for vocational advice for young people)
- www.skill.org.uk (the UK National Bureau for Students With Disabilities, which promotes opportunities for young people with disability in further education, training, and employment)
- www.euteach.com (for resources for teaching about chronic illness in adolescent health)

# 6 Health promotion

Russell Viner, Aidan Macfarlane

Health can be defined as optimum physical, emotional, social, spiritual, and intellectual health. Health promotion is the science or art of helping people change their lifestyle to move towards a state of optimal health. Lifestyle change can be facilitated through a combination of efforts to increase awareness, change behaviour, and create environments that support good health practices.

## Need for health promotion

There are five main reasons for a particular health promotion focus on young people.

**Health behaviours in youth continue into adult life**
One of the most compelling arguments for a focus on adolescent health is that adolescence is a time when new health behaviours are laid down—behaviours that track into adulthood and will influence health and morbidity throughout life. Health behaviours in childhood are dominated by parental instruction and shared family values. During adolescence young people begin to explore alternative or "adult" health behaviours, including smoking, drinking alcohol, drug misuse, violence, and sexual intimacy. The continuity of these behaviours into adulthood is well documented.

Health behaviours relating to exercise and food are also laid down in adolescence and track into adult life. Adolescent obesity predicts adult obesity, which is strongly and independently predictive of cardiovascular risk, and cardiovascular risk in young adulthood is highly related to the degree of adiposity as early as age 13 years. Evidence also shows that health in adolescence can have a considerable impact on the development of adult conditions. This evidence challenges earlier notions that adolescents moving into adulthood "grow out of" health risk behaviours and mental health problems.

**Immediate effects of adolescent health behaviours**
Adolescent health behaviours have a direct effect on immediate as well as long term health outcomes and quality of life—for example, taking exercise, engaging in risky sexual behaviour (resulting in sexually transmitted infections or teenage pregnancy), and using the roads safely.

**Worrying trends in morbidity and mortality**
Adolescent mortality and morbidity show worrying trends in national priority areas, such as mental health (for example, male suicide rates), sexual health (teenage pregnancies), and cardiovascular risk (such as obesity and diabetes). Earlier engagement in sexual activity, high rates of teenage pregnancy, and the threat of HIV have similarly focused attention on adolescents. Given the evidence on the continuity of health risk behaviours in adolescence into adulthood, morbidity trends in adolescence argue strongly for urgent attention to adolescents' health and for the development of targeted, adolescent specific interventions.

**Developmental issues**
Dynamic and continued development in every aspect of a young person's life during adolescence means that young

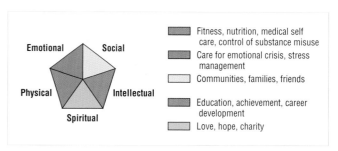

Domains for health promotion. Adapted from O'Donnell MP. *American Journal of Health Promotion* 1989;3(3)5

---

**Major health promotion areas in adolescence**
- Health risk behaviours (smoking, alcohol use, drug misuse, sexual health, and risk taking)
- Parent-adolescent communication
- Depression and mental health
- Violence
- Physical activity, nutrition, and obesity
- Health inequalities and social exclusion

---

**Prevalence of regular smoking rises from 1% at age 11 years to 24% at 15 years, and over 90% of adult smokers began smoking as teenagers; similarly, few people start experimenting with alcohol and drugs after their teenage years**

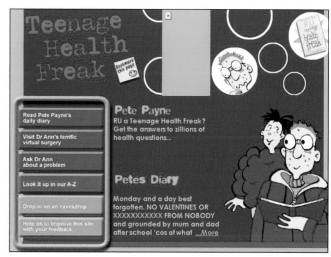

The website Teenage Health Freak (www.teenagehealthfreak.org) promotes health in a user friendly way to teenagers

**Improvements in mortality and morbidity in early childhood have not been matched in adolescence**

people have distinct needs in terms of delivery of health promotion messages.

In early adolescence, concrete thinking predominates, with young people generally able to understand only linear "concrete" relations between cause and effect. In this very literal context, messages that smoking causes lung cancer can be rejected as irrelevant, as they know that their friends who smoke do not have lung cancer.

**Health promotion messages should begin in early adolescence, as the key risk periods for starting smoking, taking drugs, and taking sexual risks are before age 14. In this early stage, health promotion messages should focus on the "here and now" risk rather than risks in adult life**

### Implications of adolescent development for health promotion in adolescence

|  | Psychological development | Social development | Implications for health promotion |
| --- | --- | --- | --- |
| Early adolescence | Concrete thinking but grasp of moral concepts; assessment and adjustment of body image | Realising difference from parents; start of strong peer group; start of health risk behaviours | Start health promotion messages, using concrete motivators; focus on "here and now"; use peer educators or role models; current physical health can be important motivator |
| Mid-adolescence | Abstract thinking develops, mainly in relation to others (self is "bullet proof") | Increasing autonomy (away from parents) | Target health promotion messages as for early adolescence; specifically address issues of risk to self as well as others |
| Late adolescence | Complex abstract thought and further development of identity and body image | Social autonomy; splitting of peer group into smaller groups and couples | Health promotion messages can address many possible outcomes of an action; targeting of messages at partners and close friends |

### Clustering of health risk

Health risk behaviours cluster in adolescence, meaning that those who smoke are also more likely to drink alcohol and take drugs. They are also more likely to engage in risky sexual behaviour and be the victims or perpetrators of violence. This is because many health problems in adolescence have important risk factors in common. Academic failure and dropping out of school (rarely attending) are associated with the development of antisocial behaviour, higher rates of substance misuse, tobacco use, and emotional problems. Similarly, the young person's mental health and patterns of family attachment are strongly associated with many important health outcomes and other established risk factors.

## Settings for health promotion

The main current strategic approaches to health promotion for adolescents have three main emphases. The first, and by far the most effective, is health promotion by society as a whole on behalf of adolescents—for example, banning cigarette advertising and making emergency contraception available over the counter.

The second is health promotion by professionals with a "health education" interest, exhorting adolescents to behave in healthy ways—for example, not to smoke, to use contraception, and to eat a balanced diet. These individual approaches are not effective. The third approach is to improve young people's social abilities. Evidence exists that improving these abilities so that young people can choose whether to accept or reject certain courses of behaviour—for example, reject a lift home by a drunken boyfriend—is also effective in enabling young people to make independent choices about individual health related behaviours. It may also improve young people's self esteem.

However, a considerable body of evidence suggests that the most effective health promotion intervention for young people would be to improve the socioeconomic circumstances in which young people are raised and to create greater socioeconomic equality in the population as a whole. Good evidence shows also that health promotion interventions at society level on behalf of adolescents (for example, increasing the price of cigarettes and banning cigarette advertising) are far more effective than health education messages directed at adolescents (for example, "don't smoke").

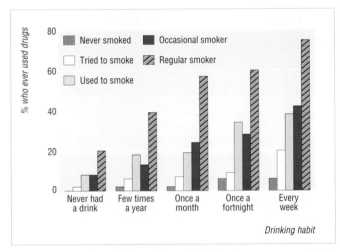

Drug use by smoking behaviour and usual drinking frequency among 11-15 year olds, England, 1998. Adapted from data from Office for National Statistics (www.ons.gov.uk)

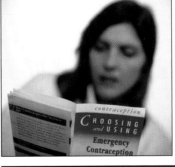

Promoting health to society as a whole (for example, making emergency contraception available over the counter) is more effective than simply urging adolescents to behave healthily

### Effective health promotion strategies

- Strategies should be on behalf of adolescents rather than directed at adolescents
- Interventions for adolescents should be simultaneous at government, community, and local level
- Interventions should focus on increasing adolescents' overall self esteem and self empowerment rather than on single health issues
- Health professionals should act as advocates on behalf of young people and as providers to young people and their carers of the most relevant and up to date evidence based information; they should use methods and language deemed appropriate by the adolescents themselves

Interventions can be delivered at various levels: the individual level, the family level, the school level, the community level, and the national level.

# Resilience

Recognising that adolescents often engage in more than one risky behaviour and that these behaviours often have common underlying predisposing factors (such as poor socioeconomic circumstances or poor mental health), evidence is growing that effective health promotion interventions for a specific risk or protective factor are both highly effective and also likely to have direct effects on a range of health outcomes.

Interventions on bullying and emotional wellbeing covering whole schools, for example, are highly effective in reducing other problems, such as smoking and drug misuse among young people.

**Levels at which interventions can be delivered**

*Individual level*—Peer interventions, including peer education; youth recreation programmes; and mentoring programmes
*Family level*—Parent training and family interventions
*School level*—Single issue, curriculum based education and "whole school" organisation and behaviour management interventions
*Community level*—Local environmental change (such as policing policy, safety issues)
*National level*—Health service reorganisation, employment and training, law and policing changes, social marketing, and socioeconomic change

**Interventions on bullying and emotional wellbeing covering whole schools can be more effective at reducing smoking than single issue smoking programmes**

**Identified risk and protective factors for adolescent health behaviours***

| Behaviour | Risk factors | Protective factors |
|---|---|---|
| Smoking | Depression and other mental health problems; alcohol use; disconnectedness from school or family; difficulty talking with parents; minority ethnicity; low school achievement; peer smoking | Family connectedness; perceived healthiness; higher parental expectations; low prevalence of smoking in school |
| Alcohol and drug misuse | Depression and other mental health problems; low self esteem; easy family access to alcohol; working outside school; difficulty talking with parents; risk factors for transition from occasional to regular substance misuse (smoking, availability of substances, peer use, other risk behaviours) | Connectedness with school and family; religious affiliation |
| Teenage pregnancy | Deprivation; city residence; low educational expectations; lack of access to sexual health services; drug and alcohol use | Connectedness with school and family; religious affiliation |
| Sexually transmitted infections | Mental health problems; substance misuse | Connectedness with school and family; religious affiliation |

*Adapted from McIntosh N, Helms P, Smyth R, eds. *Forfar and Arneil's textbook of paediatrics.* 6th ed. Edinburgh: Churchill Livingstone, 2003:1757-68

# Role of individual health workers

Despite the low efficacy of most health promotion messages at individual level, health professionals do have a role in health promotion in their clinical interactions with young people. Brief health promotion discussions about smoking during routine general practice visits can reduce smoking rates, although messages are more effective if targeted at patients who are contemplating change. The "stages of change" model of behaviour change suggests that "action oriented" advice for those who are not ready to change is at best unhelpful and could even entrench unhealthy behaviour.

Patients themselves report that health promotion advice from their doctor is best received if it takes account of their receptiveness, is conveyed in a respectful tone, avoids preaching, shows support and caring, and shows understanding of them as unique individuals.

When teenagers are seen in primary care, particular areas for health promotion are sexual health, smoking, and drug misuse. Most young people who experiment with drugs do not consult their doctor, and most doctors know less about illegal drugs than young people. Evidence from randomised trials suggests, however, that providing young people aged 11 to 13 with information about illegal drugs delays the start of drug misuse.

**Stages of change**

- Precontemplation (not yet acknowledging that there is a problem behaviour that needs to be changed)
- Contemplation (acknowledging a problem but not yet ready (or sure of wanting) to make change)
- Preparation/determination (getting ready to change)
- Action/willpower (changing behaviour)
- Maintenance (maintaining behaviour change)
- Relapse (reverting to older behaviour and abandoning new changes)

**Further reading and resources**

- Toumbourou J, Patton GC, Sawyer S, Olsson C, Webb-Pullman J, Catalano R, et al. *Evidence based health promotion. No 2. Adolescent health.* Melbourne, Australia: Department of Human Services, 2000.
- www.hda-online.org.uk/evidence/ (the Health Development Agency's "evidence base"—a searchable database of evidence on health promotion).
- www.teenagehealthfreak.org and www.lifebytes.gov.uk (teenage friendly websites that provide health promotion material for young people).

The photograph is published with permission from Damien Lovegrove.

# 7 Sexual health, contraception, and teenage pregnancy

John Tripp, Russell Viner

Sexual health becomes a new health priority in early adolescence. The sexual health of young people is a matter of intense public concern. The adverse consequences of unsafe sexual behaviour—such as pregnancy and sexually transmitted infections (STIs), including HIV infection—affect adolescents as well as adults. "Risk taking" behaviours are common when adolescents start being sexually intimate and are often linked with other health risk behaviours, such as substance misuse.

## Relationships and sexual behaviour

The median age for first sexual intercourse in the United Kingdom dropped during the early 1990s and is now stable at around 16 years for both men and women. The disparity between the sexes observed in the early 1990s has diminished. Before the age of 15, about 18% of boys and 15% of girls report having had full sexual intercourse, with similar proportions having engaged in oral sex.

Having sex for the first time at an early age is often associated with unsafe sex, in part through lack of knowledge, lack of access to contraception, lack of skills and self efficacy to negotiate contraception, having sex while drunk or stoned, or inadequate self efficacy to resist pressure.

About 10% of boys in the United Kingdom report that they were drunk or stoned when they first had sex, and 11% of girls report being pressurised by their partner when they first had sex. Of those under 16 years who have ever had sex, about a third to a half of both sexes report ever having had unsafe sex.

## Sexually transmitted infections

Considerable rises in the incidence of STIs, particularly chlamydia, have led to a major public health problem in the United Kingdom. Although rates in the under 16s have remained low, rates in 16-19 year olds and 20-24 year olds almost trebled in men and more than doubled in women during 1995 to 2001. Some studies suggest that 30-40% of sexually active teenage girls in high risk groups are infected.

Gonorrhoea, and to a lesser extent genital herpes, has shown similar increases in incidence. The highest rates of STIs are among black Caribbean and black African young people, suggesting that cultural and socioeconomic factors play a major role in the risk of acquiring and in protection against STIs.

Clinical presentations of STIs in adolescents are similar to those in adults. It is important to note that chlamydia, often asymptomatic in older adolescent girls and women, usually presents with a vaginal discharge in young adolescent girls.

---

**Risk factors for sexually transmitted infections in adolescence**

- Unsafe sex
- Multiple, sequential sexual partners
- Concurrent partners
- Mental health problems
- Concurrent substance misuse
- Physiological immaturity (chlamydia seems to easily infect the immature cervix, making teenage girls more susceptible to infection than adults)

---

**Teenagers assess and evaluate risk differently from adults and health professionals: they would rather reduce their risk of being excluded from the "in-group" or of looking immature than take notice of any perceived health risks**

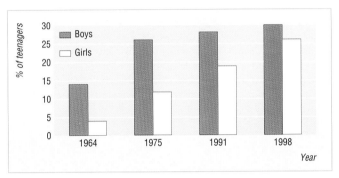

Proportion of UK teenagers who first had sexual intercourse by age 16 years, 1964-98

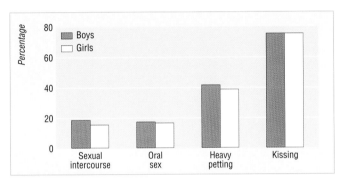

Percentages of 14 year olds in Scotland engaging in various sexual activities

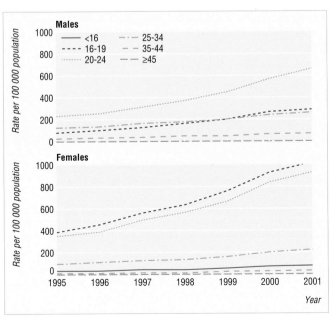

Rates of uncomplicated chlamydia infections in United Kingdom by age, 1995-2001

Early detection and treatment of curable STIs, such as chlamydia, can reduce the risk of further complications, such as infertility and ectopic pregnancy. With the easy availability of highly sensitive new nucleic acid amplification tests on voided urine, current UK recommendations support the opportunistic screening of all sexually active adolescent females attending general practice surgeries and genitourinary medicine and family planning clinics, regardless of whether they have symptoms. Screening young men without symptoms remains more controversial, although many suggest opportunistic screening similar to that provided for young women.

# Teenage pregnancy

The incidence of teenage pregnancy across Europe varies considerably. The United Kingdom has the highest rate in western Europe and is lower only than Bulgaria, Russia, and Ukraine in Europe as a whole. Throughout most of western Europe, teenage birth rates fell during the 1970s, '80s, and '90s, but in the United Kingdom, rates have remained high—at or above the level of the early '80s.

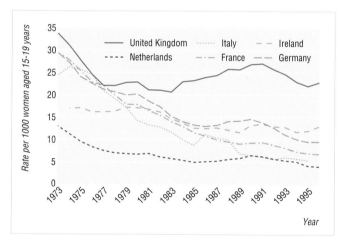

Live birth rate to women aged 15-19 years, 1973-96

It is important to recognise that for some young women, particularly from certain ethnic or social groups, teenage pregnancy can be a positive life choice. Rates of teenage pregnancy within marriage are high, for example, in some South Asian ethnic groups in the United Kingdom. However, for many other young women, the costs of teenage pregnancy can be very high, particularly when linked with poverty. These risks include poorer outcomes for the children of teenage mothers as well as for the mothers themselves.

Infant mortality among babies of teenage mothers is about 60% higher than among the babies of older mothers. These infants are also more likely to have lower birth weights, have childhood accidents, and be admitted to hospital during childhood. In the longer term, the daughters of teenage mothers are more likely to become teenage mothers themselves.

Prevention of unwanted teenage pregnancies is a high priority in many countries. In the United Kingdom, strategies are based on the cycles of social exclusion and disadvantage that both cause and follow teenage pregnancy.

High quality evidence shows that health promotion behavioural programmes using peer educators of a similar age reduce the prevalence of sexual activity at age 16 years. Although programmes that promote abstinence have a logical appeal, no high quality studies have shown the effectiveness of such approaches, and such programmes are not seen as

---

## Clinical features of sexually transmitted infections in adolescents

### Chlamydia
- No symptoms in half of males and 70% of females
- Vaginal discharge is usual presentation in girls aged under 13 years
- Pelvic inflammatory disease can be asymptomatic

### Gonorrhoea
- No symptoms in up to 80% of females
- Urethritis and discharge is common in males
- Girls aged under 13 years usually have vaginal discharge
- Pharyngeal and rectal infections may be present

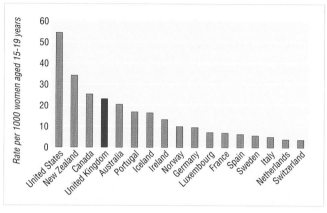

Births per 1000 women aged 15-19 years, 1998

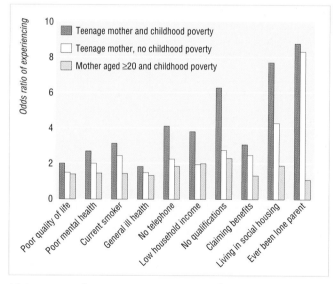

Adult outcomes of teenage pregnancy compared with a reference level for women who give birth at age 23-32 and had no childhood poverty

---

**Factors known to protect young people from teenage pregnancy include higher levels of connectedness with school and family; long term, stable relationship with a partner; and strong religious beliefs**

---

## Risk factors for teenage pregnancy

- Poverty (the strongest risk factor)
- Looked-after children (children "in care")
- Children of teenage mothers
- Low educational achievement
- Poor transition from school to work at age 16 years
- Sexual abuse
- Mental health problems
- Crime

acceptable by many teenagers or professionals as they potentially limit young peoples' rights and autonomy.

# Contraception

In the United Kingdom about 75% of young people in early adolescence and 85% in mid-adolescence, of both sexes, have reported that they used an effective form of contraception the last time they had sex.

Teenagers are relatively poor users of both barrier and hormonal contraceptives. Condoms remain the contraceptive of choice of young people; over 75% reported that they used condoms at their last sexual intercourse (15% reported using the oral contraceptive, 1% injectable contraception, and 6% emergency contraception).

The first time a young person has sex is one of the riskiest times for young people in the United Kingdom: half of the under 16s and a third of those aged 16-19 use no contraception the first time they have sex, as much as double the rates in other developed countries, including the United States.

---

### Proportion of adolescents using contraception at first intercourse

*Netherlands*—85% of "young people"
*Denmark*—80% of 15-16 year olds
*Switzerland*—80% of "adolescents"
*United States*—78% of "adolescents"
*France*—74% of "girls"; 79% of "boys"
*New Zealand*—75% of "sexually active teenagers"
*United Kingdom*—50% of under 16s; 66% of 16-19 year olds

---

Health promotion targeted at teenagers and the provision of free condoms improves contraceptive use by teenagers. The most appropriate contraceptives for most young people are likely to be condoms and the contraceptive pill. However, teenagers have a relatively high failure rate with both these methods because of "technical problems" (condom failure and irregular use of the pill). Because of this, some countries are promoting the "double Dutch" method—using condoms plus oral contraception to protect against both pregnancy and STIs.

Emergency contraception is not a substitute for a regular form of contraception and does not protect against STIs. Access to emergency contraception, however, is an important and effective preventive measure against an unwanted pregnancy. In the United Kingdom, knowledge of emergency contraception is low among young people—for example, less than half know about the 72 hour "window of opportunity." Young women aged 16 and over can obtain emergency contraception over the counter at pharmacies. However, for girls under age 16, such contraception is available only on prescription (either from doctors or, in exceptional circumstances, from approved pharmacists), thus imposing substantial limitations on its use by young teenagers at risk.

Good evidence to support current practice is limited. Increasing numbers of people believe that campaigns and educational programmes that promote postponement or temporary abstinence much more strongly than the current British programmes do might result in greater health benefits. ABC programmes (Abstinence, Be faithful, and if not, use a Condom) seem to have been remarkably successful compared with promotion of barrier contraception in some African countries, and the politically driven "abstinence-only" campaigns in the United States have coincided with falls in teenage pregnancy rates without the increases in STIs seen in the United Kingdom.

---

### Factors that reduce rates of teenage pregnancy

- Adequate sex education and information
- Health promotion targeted at teenagers (advising that they consider whether they are ready for intercourse and encouraging the use of barrier and combined barrier and hormonal contraception)
- Sexual health services that are "adolescent friendly"
- Postponement of sexual activity
- "Life option" programmes to give alternatives to early parenting
- Assertiveness training and communication about contraception
- Problem solving and decision making skills
- Improving family communication about sex

---

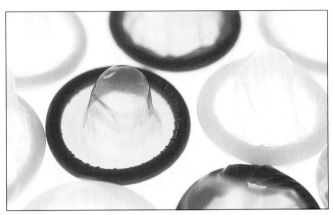

Condoms remain the contraceptive of choice of young people, though the combined use of condoms plus the contraceptive pill is probably the most effective option

---

### Promoting contraception in primary care

- Make condoms easily available without the need for counselling or appointments
- Ensure that health promotion materials cover emergency contraception and young people's legal rights to contraception in general
- Ensure that materials are displayed where they will be read
- Offer contraceptive methods that are attractive to young people (such as not stigmatising), useable just at the time of intercourse, and cheap and easily obtainable
- Advise use of "double Dutch" method of contraception

---

### Guidance from UK Department of Health*

A doctor or other health professional providing contraceptive advice or treatment to someone aged under 16 without parental consent should be satisfied that:

- The young person will understand the advice and the moral, social, and emotional implications
- The young person cannot be persuaded to tell their parents or allow the doctor to tell them that they are seeking contraceptive advice
- The young person is having, or is likely to have, unprotected sex whether they receive the advice or not
- The young person's physical or mental health is likely to deteriorate unless they receive the advice or treatment
- It is in the young person's best interests to give contraceptive advice or treatment without parental consent

*Adapted from Department of Health. *Best practice guidelines for doctors and other health professionals on the provision of advice and treatment to young people under 16 on contraception, sexual and reproductive health.* 2004. www.dh.gov.uk (search for: 3382)

---

**Evidence is increasing that, although abstinence campaigns may delay young people's first sexual intercourse, they may also increase their risk of having unprotected sex when they do begin having sex**

# Providing sexual health services to adolescents

Sexual health services for young people must be available in general practice in addition to specialist services. A recent study reported that over 90% of pregnant teenagers had discussed contraception with their general practitioner in the year before becoming pregnant, confirming primary care as the main provider of health services. Those at risk of pregnancy are also at risk of STIs, and it would be logical to provide both contraceptive and STI testing services together.

Siting of services may be critical. Because of reluctance about being identified as using a sexual health service, young people may prefer to attend a general primary care clinic rather than a specialist service, even if the primary care clinic is not as youth friendly. The sex of the health professional also seems to be important, with a tendency for primary care or family planning services to be used by young women, while young men may simply buy condoms from pharmacies or vending machines.

Providing sexual health and contraceptive services in an "age appropriate" environment and manner is particularly important for adolescents, as they will simply not use services they regard as inaccessible or unfriendly. Young people report that confidentiality, a non-judgmental approach, informality, accessibility, and the ability to choose whether they see a male or female health worker are the most important factors in deciding whether to use services.

## Further reading and resources

- Rogstad KE, Ahmed-Jushuf IH, Robinson AJ. Standards for comprehensive sexual health services for young people under 25 years: UK national survey. *Int J STD AIDS* 2002;13:420-4.
- Social Exclusion Unit. *Teenage pregnancy report.* London: Stationery Office, 1999.
- Toumbourou J, Patton GC, Sawyer S, Olsson C, Webb-Pullman J, Catalano R, et al. *Evidence based health promotion. No 2. Adolescent health.* Melbourne: Department of Human Services, Victoria, 2000.
- Trust for the Study of Adolescence. *Key data on adolescence.* Brighton: TSA, 2003.

The first graph is adapted from Coleman and Schofield (*Key data on adolescence.* Brighton: Trust for the Study of Adolescence, 2003). The graph showing the sexual practices of Scottish 14 year olds is adapted from Todd J et al (*Health behaviours of Scottish schoolchildren. Sexual health in the 1990s.* Edinburgh: University of Edinburgh, 1999). The graph showing rates of chlamydia infection is adapted from PHLS, 2001. The graphs showing births per 1000 women, live birth rates, and adult outcomes and the box on contraception at first intercourse are adapted from the Social Exclusion Unit's *Teenage Pregnancy Report* (see "Further reading" box). The photograph of the condoms is published with permission from RESO/Rex and the cartoon on this page with permission from IPPF/BBC.

## Desirable features of sexual health services for adolescents

- Confidentiality
- Knowledge about the legal framework covering services to adolescents
- Good access (the setting and the approach of staff should be adolescent friendly; services should allow self referral; they should be close to areas used by young people and be accessible by public transport; after-school and/or weekend sessions should be available)
- "Men only" clinics as well as clinics for females
- Non-judgmental attitudes
- Choice of staff by gender where possible
- Awareness of cultural issues (particularly in relation to Asian ethnicities)
- Contraceptive methods appropriate to age of young person
- Free and on-site provision of treatment for sexually transmitted infections
- Counselling services appropriate for young people
- Clear routes of referral to and liaison with specialist services (including genitourinary medicine, child health professionals, and social services)

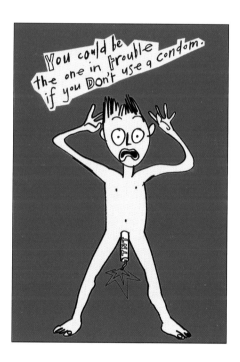

# 8 Substance misuse: alcohol, tobacco, inhalants, and other drugs

Yvonne Bonomo, Jenny Proimos

Misuse of alcohol, tobacco, inhalants, and other drugs is now widespread among adolescents internationally and causes substantial health problems in this group. This article explores the misuse of these substances.

## Epidemiology

Alcohol and tobacco are by far the most commonly used substances by young people and result in 95% of morbidity and mortality related to substance misuse in this age group. Despite the public and political concerns about use of illicit drugs, such drugs are much less commonly used than alcohol and tobacco, although they may pose more serious immediate health risks. The "gateway" theory about drugs (that tobacco and alcohol may lead on to use of illicit drugs) does not always hold in adolescence. Although it is true that almost all users of illicit drugs have used tobacco and alcohol, most adolescents who regularly use tobacco and alcohol do not progress to using illicit drugs.

### Alcohol

Alcohol consumption typically begins in adolescence. About a fifth of 12-13 year olds report drinking alcohol; the proportion increases to 40-50% by age 14-15 and to over 70% by age 17. In the United Kingdom the proportion of adolescents reporting weekly drinking has changed little over the past 15 years. On average, about 40% of young people report binge drinking; the main reasons given for bingeing are enjoyment and the fact that the alcohol helps them to be more sociable.

### Smoking

The proportion of young people who smoke regularly rises from about 1% at age 11 years to 26% of girls and 21% of boys at age 15 in the United Kingdom. Overall, smoking rates among young people have changed little in the past 20 years, although rates among girls overtook those among boys from the mid-1980s.

### Drugs

Cannabis is the most common drug of misuse in Western countries. Cannabis use usually starts at about 16-17 years old, with 30-50% of this age group reporting that they have at least tried cannabis. Regular use, however, is less common, with about 10% of adolescents reporting weekly use and about 3% daily use.

**Throughout the article, when the term substance misuse is used, it refers to the whole group of substances (alcohol, tobacco, inhalants, and other drugs)**

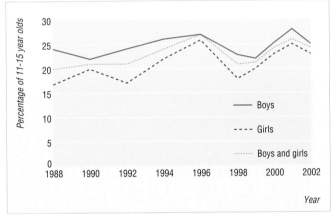

Proportions of 11-15 year olds in England who reported drinking during preceding week, 1988-2002. Adapted from Boreham et al. *Smoking, drinking and drug use among young people*. London: Stationery Office, 2002

---

**Classification of harmful drugs in United Kingdom**

*Class A drugs*—Opiates such as diamorphine (heroin), dipipanone, pethidine, morphine; powerful stimulants such as cocaine and its derivative "crack"; hallucinogens such as lysergide (LSD) and mescaline; methylated amphetamines such as methylenedioxymethamphetamine (MDMA, ecstasy); methadone

*Class B drugs*—Amphetamine (sniffed or smoked); dihydocodeine (DF118); methylphenobarbitone

*Class C drugs*—Benzodiazapines such as diazepam, temazepam, chlordiazepoxide, and nitrazepam; cannabis resin

Class A drugs are the most harmful; class B are harmful but less harmful than class A; class C are potentially harmful when misused. Any class B drug prepared for injection becomes class A

---

**Adverse effects of cannabis misuse**

- Social, interpersonal, and legal difficulties
- Cognitive impairment, including memory problems
- Effects on respiratory system (such as chronic bronchitis, increased susceptibility to pneumonia, and possibly an increased risk of lung carcinoma)
- Increased risk of psychosis
- Cannabis dependence (occurs in about 10% of heavy users)

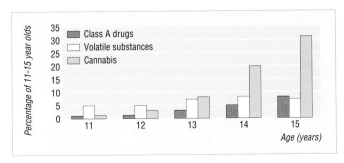

Percentage of 11-15 year olds in England who used drugs during preceding year, by type of drug and age, 2002. Class A drugs are heroin, methadone, cocaine, ecstasy, LSD, injected amphetamines. Boreham et al. *Smoking, drinking and drug use among young people*. London: Stationery Office, 2002

**Desired and adverse effects of class A drugs and their administration route**

| Drug | Desired effects | Adverse effects |
|---|---|---|
| Amphetamines (sniffed or injected) | Increased self confidence and capacity for concentration; heightened alertness | Jaw clenching; teeth grinding; difficulty concentrating; dehydration; cardiac arrhythmias; sudden death |
| Ecstasy (oral) | Positive mood; feelings of intimacy; euphoria; increased energy | As for amphetamines |
| Cocaine (snorted, smoked, injected intravenously) | Positive mood; euphoria; increased energy | Muscle twitching; dizziness; confusion; anxiety and paranoia; acute myocardial infarction; cardiomyopathy; cardiac arrhythmias; cocaine psychosis; violent or aggressive behaviour; cocaine dependence syndrome |
| Opiates (such as heroin; burned, snorted, injected intravenously) | Euphoria; wellbeing; sedative effects | Venous collapse; abscesses; heart and other major organ damage; opiate dependence syndrome; respiratory depression; death |

## Inhalants

Prevalence estimates vary, but as many as 5% of young adolescents in the general population may be misusing paint, glue, or petrol. This form of substance misuse is most common among younger high risk adolescents, as these substances are readily available and their purchase and possession are not illegal.

## Trajectories of substance misuse

Not all young people who experiment with substances proceed to levels that bring health problems. Some use certain substances for recreational purposes, whereas others use them for self medication (for example, for insomnia or emotional distress). Recurrent problems related to substance misuse (such as difficulties with family or friends and school attendance) most commonly arise as a result of increased frequency of high dose use. A minority of adolescents with problematic high dose use progress to clinical harm and dependence.

## Risk factors

A number of individual and environmental factors influence substance misuse by adolescents. Many of them "cluster" within an individual. Consideration of protective as well as risk factors is clinically useful, both in the assessment of risk in a young person and in the development of a management plan.

## Assessing substance misuse

### Establishing rapport

Successful work with adolescents, including dealing with their substance misuse, requires the development of a trusting relationship and good rapport, particularly in terms of confidentiality. In allowing the young person to participate in management options, the practitioner also needs to feel confident that the young person understands the consequences of his or her health choices.

### Taking a history

In primary care, specific screening questionnaires for substance misuse have not been shown to be any more effective than taking a broad medical and psychosocial history. A psychosocial history includes information about the social, cultural,

**When vaporised and inhaled, paint, glue, and petrol rapidly result in intoxication and euphoria**

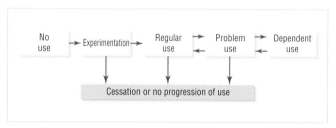

It is important with adolescents to consider where he or she lies in the spectrum of misuse

**Risk and protective factors for substance misuse in adolescents**

*Biological factors*—Alterations in the enzymes involved in the metabolic pathways of substances; alterations in genetic expression of central nervous system receptors mediating substance effects

*Temperament and personality traits*—Antisocial personality disorder; sensation seeking trait

*Familial factors*—Familial attitudes that are favourable to the use of substances; parental modelling of substance misuse; poor or inconsistent parenting practices

*Early onset of substance use*—Individuals who report drinking before the age of 15, for example, are about four times more likely to develop alcohol dependence than those who delay starting drinking until young adulthood

*Emotional and behavioural problems*—Conduct disorder; depression; attention-deficit/hyperactivity disorder

*Poor social connections*—To school and to community groups, for example

*Peer use of substances*—This is one of the strongest predictors of substance misuse in young people

**Non-specific signs of substance misuse**

*Physical complaints*—Increased fatigue, repeated unexplained health complaints

*Emotional changes*—Friends or relatives noting personality change; onset of lowered mood; lack of interest in usual activities; withdrawal from family; sudden changes in mood

*Social problems*—Irresponsible behaviour; decline in school performance, attendance, or conduct; more time spent with new friends who are less interested in standard home and school activities; legal complications; increased need for money

educational, and vocational background of the adolescent as well as potential mental health problems. As concurrent misuse of more than one substance is common among adolescents, it is important to ask specifically about each substance, including alcohol and tobacco. A urine screen may be a useful tool to assess the range of substances used in the previous days.

---

**Specific signs of substance misuse**

*Intravenous drug habit*—Pupil constriction (opiates); venepuncture marks and old scars (on cubital fossa, forearm, lower limb, or neck)
*Inhalant misuse*—Paint stains on clothing and skin (particularly around mouth and nose and on hands); chemicals smelt on breath
*Withdrawal effects*—Agitation, tremor, tachycardia, or dilated pupils (associated with some drugs, such as opiates)

---

### History and physical examination in assessment of substance misuse in adolescents

| General areas | Specific issues |
|---|---|
| *History (also explore reason for presentation)* | |
| Substance misuse | Ask about quantity, frequency, typical pattern of use, age of starting, time of most recent use, administration |
| Risk behaviours related to substance misuse | Ask about frequency of intoxication, bingeing, overdosing, driving habits, unsafe sex, sharing needles |
| Development of tolerance | Ask adolescent if he or she needs more of the substance now, compared with before, to achieve same effect |
| Complications related to substance misuse | Ask about hepatitis B and C; HIV; liver disease; seizures (if so, when using substance or when withdrawing from it?); cardiac problems |
| Psychiatric history | Ask about depression and anxiety, insomnia, hallucinations, paranoia, self harm and suicide attempts, schizophrenia, and drug induced psychosis |
| Social history | Ask about support, relationships, living environment, education and employment, legal complications of substance misuse, family history of substance misuse |
| *Examination* | |
| Evidence of intoxication? | Alcohol: alcohol on breath, blood alcohol concentration, sedated, slurred speech, or ataxic gait? Opiates: pinpoint pupils, low blood pressure, or venepuncture marks? Benzodiazepines: disinhibited or intoxicated but not drunk? Psychostimulants: rapid speech, large pupils, agitation, restlessness, or high blood pressure? |
| Evidence of withdrawal? | Alcohol: tremulous, or high blood pressure? Opiates: dilated pupils, high blood pressure, sweaty, rhinorrhoea, or cramps? Benzodiazepines: tremulous, hyper-reflexia, depersonalisation, hypersensitivity? Psychostimulants: agitation or restlessness? |
| Other observations | Underweight, anaemic, jaundiced, or splinter haemorrhages in nailbeds? Intravenous drug use: injection sites (present, absent; new, old), cellulitis, abscesses, or thrombophlebitis? Inhalants: paint on fingers? Smell of solvent on the breath? |
| Other disorders | Respiratory infection, endocarditis (especially right sided), hepatomegaly, mental health problems and neurological disorders (peripheral neuropathy, ataxia) secondary to alcohol or inhalant misuse? |

---

### Assessing dependence

It is important to identify when the substance misuse has led to dependence and when it has not. Dependence is likely when the young person experiences *(a)* difficulty controlling (that is, limiting) use of the substance despite considerable negative consequences; *(b)* tolerance to the substance, needing increasing amounts to get the same effect; and *(c)* withdrawal symptoms when not using that substance.

---

**Preventing substance misuse by adolescents**

- Substance misuse by adolescents is shaped by several factors including the economic, physical, and social environment
- Narrowly focused short term interventions, such as mass media campaigns, have been largely ineffective in adolescents
- Programmes are more likely to succeed if they take a long term perspective; encourage acquisition of skills; promote social inclusion; and are appropriate developmentally for young people

---

## Managing substance misuse

Helping a young person to reduce or stop substance misuse requires patience, an open minded and non-judgmental approach, and an understanding of the stages of change in human behaviour. Doctors can help facilitate change, but only the individual can change his or her behaviour.

### Stages of change

Behaviour change takes time. Change passes through several stages that have been well described (Prochaska, 1991; see Further Reading box).

Many young people who smoke tobacco or who often have drinking binges have not seriously considered changing. Consultations therefore can involve general discussion with the young person about his or her smoking or drinking, without

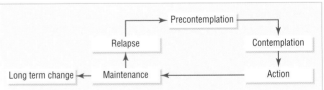

**Precontemplation** No serious thought about behaviour change in next six months
**Contemplation** Serious thought about changing an unhealthy behaviour (but not yet taking action)
**Action** Overt modification of behaviour
**Maintenance** Period after overt behaviour change until the behaviour stops or person relapses

Keeping in mind the process of change is integral to working with adolescents

the assumption or expectation that there will be an immediate change in current pattern of misuse. Motivational conversations about the benefits and risks of change provide important opportunities for advising young people what the potential harms of substance misuse are, how to recognise escalating use, and which strategies are useful for avoiding these adverse outcomes. This can help young people to move from the precontemplation stage to the contemplation stage.

## Treatment options

Once the young person decides to take action on his or her substance misuse, options for management include *(a)* counselling, including brief therapy such as cognitive behaviour therapy; *(b)* drug withdrawal or "detoxification" either in a residential setting or as an outpatient; *(c)* pharmacotherapy (preferably after consultation with a drug and alcohol specialist); and *(d)* rehabilitation through an outpatient programme or in a residential setting. These interventions are used in varying ways and in differing contexts of substance misuse in young people. It has not yet been clearly established which strategy or approach is the best. Harm reduction strategies, which aim to minimise harm while reducing use, are an important part of the overall strategy to reduce drug related harm.

## Comorbidities of substance misuse

As well as working with the young person to move him or her towards reduced substance misuse, primary healthcare practitioners need to monitor medical issues—from nutrition and sexually transmitted diseases to HIV screening and mental health concerns.

## Setting realistic expectations

Managing substance misuse in adolescents requires patience because complex behaviours and emotions take time to change and usually follow a fluctuating course, with frequent relapses. Positive reinforcement through comments on any change in substance misuse behaviour, however small, can be valuable in continuing to motivate the individual.

This is particularly important in the context of relapses. Substance misuse usually follows a chronic relapsing course, yet relapses are rarely anticipated. Some young people may expect one admission to a detoxification unit to be sufficient to "cure" them of their drug habit. Reassurance that relapse is normal reduces the sense of failure that potentially undermines any motivation to continue.

Reminding the adolescent of previous successes and exploring with them what they understand to be the cause of the relapse is important. This may help them to understand patterns in their behaviour, which they can modify in the future. In cases of severe substance dependence, medically supervised withdrawal followed by rehabilitation, either in a residential setting or as an intensive outpatient programme, are indicated.

## Reintegration

An important part of managing chronic substance misuse includes reintegration into education and employment and into healthier alternatives to substance misuse, such as sport and other activities or hobbies.

The photograph is reproduced with permission from Sutton-Hibbert/Rex.

## Topics for motivational conversations in drug and alcohol work with young people

Increasing motivation to change and therefore progress from precontemplation to contemplation can occur through exploring:
- The advantages and disadvantages of the misuse (for example, "Drinking can make you feel relaxed and at ease in company, but sometimes being drunk can be an ugly look. What is your experience?")
- The factors that bother them most about potential behaviour change (for example, girls often worry that they will gain weight if they stop smoking)
- Their reactions to the adverse consequences of which they are currently at risk (for example, unwanted pregnancy or sexually transmitted disease through having had unsafe sex while intoxicated)

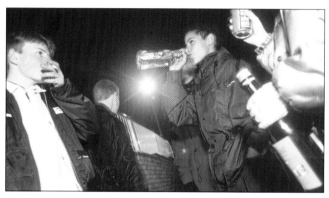

Harm reduction strategies may include encouraging moderation as well as abstinence; providing information on safe levels of alcohol consumption; advising on hazards of drinking and driving; providing information on health risks of drugs; advising not to share needles; and giving phone helplines and and other information sources

## Further reading

- Hawkins JD, Catalano RF, Miller JY. Risk and protective factors for alcohol and other drug problems in adolescence and early adulthood: implications for substance abuse prevention. *Psychol Bull* 1992;112:64-105.
- Prochaska JO. Assessing how people change. *Cancer* 1991;67:805-7.
- Kandel D, Logan J. Patterns of drug use from adolescence to young adulthood: I. Periods of risk for initiation, continued use, and discontinuation. *Am J Public Health* 1984;74:660-6.
- Yamaguchi K, Kandel DB. Patterns of drug use from adolescence to young adulthood: II. Sequences of progression. *Am J Public Health* 1984;74:668-72.
- Joint Working Party of the Royal College of Physicians and the British Paediatric Association. *Alcohol and the young.* London: RCP, 1995.
- Goldenring JM, Cohen E. Getting into adolescent heads. *Contemporary Paediatrics* 1988;5:75.

# 9 Common mental health problems

Pierre-André Michaud, Eric Fombonne

The World Health Organization defines mental health as a "state of well-being whereby individuals recognize their abilities, are able to cope with the normal stresses of life, work productively and fruitfully, and make a contribution to their communities." Applying such adult based definitions to adolescents and identifying mental health problems in young people can be difficult, given the substantial changes in behaviour, thinking capacities, and identity that occur during the teenage years. The impact of changing youth subcultures on behaviour and priorities can also make it difficult to define mental health and mental health problems in adolescents. Although mental disorders reflect psychiatric disturbance, adolescents may be affected more broadly by mental health problems. These include various difficulties and burdens that interfere with adolescent development and adversely affect quality of life emotionally, socially, and vocationally.

Mental disorders and mental health problems seem to have increased considerably among adolescents in the past 20-30 years. The rise has been driven by social change, including disruption of family structure, growing youth unemployment, and increasing educational and vocational pressures. The prevalence of mental health disorders among 11 to 15 year olds in Great Britain is estimated to be 11%, with conduct problems more common among boys and depression and anxiety more common among girls.

The identification, treatment, and follow up of mental health problems in young people can be complicated. Parents and teachers may dismiss problems as merely reflecting adolescent turmoil. Young people are often very reluctant to seek help, owing to developmental needs about being "normal" at the time when they are exploring identity issues and trying to engage with a peer group.

## Normal behaviour versus mental problems

Variations of mood and temporary deviant behaviours are part of the normal adolescent process. It is normal for young people to feel depressed from time to time and for this mood to last several days. Similarly, many young people will experiment with drugs or "delinquent" behaviours as part of normal exploration of their own identity. Such normal behaviours can be distinguished from more serious problems by the duration, persistence, and impact of the symptoms.

### Symptoms needing assessment

- Signs of overt mood depression (low mood, tearfulness, lack of interest in usual activities)
- Somatic complaints such as headache, stomach ache, backache, and sleep problems
- Self harming behaviours
- Aggression
- Isolation and loneliness
- Deviant behaviour such as theft and robbery
- Change in school performance or behaviour
- Use of psychoactive substances, including over the counter medications
- Weight loss or failure to gain weight with growth

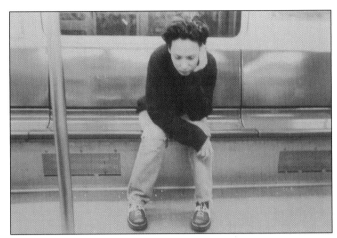

Mental health problems can affect adolescents' quality of life

### Definition of a mental disorder*

A mental disorder:
- Is behavioural or psychological
- Is of clinical significance
- Is accompanied by a concomitant distress and/or a raised risk of death, or an important loss of freedom
- Involves an unexpected cultural response to any situation

*World Health Organization, 2003 (see "Further Reading" box)

### Mental health problems and disorders in adolescents*

| Problem or disorder | Prevalence (%) |
| --- | --- |
| *Common* | |
| Depression | 3-5 |
| Anxiety | 4-6 |
| Attention-deficit/hyperactivity disorder | 2-4 |
| Eating disorders | 1-2 |
| Conduct disorder | 4-6 |
| Substance misuse disorder | 2-3 |
| *Less common* | |
| Panic disorder | 1-2 |
| Post-traumatic stress disorder | 1-2 |
| Borderline personality disorder | 1-3 |
| Schizophrenia | 0.5 |
| Autistic spectrum disorders (such as autism, Asperger's syndrome) | 0.6 |

*Costello et al (*Arch Gen Psychiatry* 2003;60:837-44); Ford et al (*J Am Acad Child Adolesc Psychiatry* 2003;42:1203-11); Fombonne (*J Autism Dev Disord* 2003;33:365-82).

### Criteria for distinguishing normal variations in behaviour from more serious problems

*Duration*—Consider as potentially harmful any problems that last more than a few weeks; reassess mental state on several occasions
*Persistence and severity of fixed symptoms*—Loss of normal fluctuations in mood and behaviour
*Impact of symptoms*—School work, interpersonal relations, home and leisure activities

Assessing young people's risk in non-mental health settings in primary or secondary care can be difficult. Basic requisites include a non-judgmental approach that recognises the young person's rights to confidentiality, where appropriate for the level of risk involved. Several validated screening questionnaires can be used to assess the risk of serious mental health problems in adolescents (Hack et al, "Further reading" box).

# Depression

The recognition, evaluation, and treatment of depression and related suicidal or self harming behaviour are the highest priorities in adolescent mental health. Epidemiological studies suggest that at any one time 8% to 10% of adolescents have severe depression. This means that the major burden of assessing and managing adolescent depression falls on primary care practitioners.

---

**Signs and symptoms of severe depression\***

- Persistent sad or irritable mood
- Loss of interest in activities once enjoyed
- Substantial change in appetite or body weight
- Oversleeping or difficulty sleeping
- Psychomotor agitation or retardation
- Loss of energy
- Feelings of worthlessness or inappropriate guilt
- Difficulty concentrating
- Recurrent thoughts of death or suicide

*Five or more of these symptoms (including at least one of the first two) must persist for two or more weeks before major depression can be diagnosed*

*World Health Organization (see "Further Reading" box)

---

Adolescence sees the transition from childhood depressive illnesses (depression rare, male predominance, symptoms masked) to more adult forms, with a much increased incidence, a female predominance, and a greater likelihood of presenting with depressed mood. However, masked presentations (for example, behavioural problems, substance misuse, school phobia or failure at school, fatigue, and other somatic symptoms) remain common in early adolescence, particularly in boys.

To evaluate risk of depression properly, young people must be interviewed confidentially and additional information gathered from parents as well as other sources (such as teachers, social workers, or youth workers). As well as eliciting symptoms and risk factors for depression, it is essential to assess potential suicide risk in depressed young people. They must be asked about past and present suicidal ideation and self harming behaviour, past attempts, and whether they plan to harm themselves. Asking about suicide reduces rather than increases the risk of suicide.

Treatment usually involves psychotherapy, drug treatment, and a mixture of measures directed at improving the home and school environment.

# School phobia

School phobia, also called school refusal, is defined as a persistent and irrational fear of going to school. It must be distinguished from a mere dislike of school that is related to issues such as a new teacher, a difficult examination, the class bully, lack of confidence, or having to undress for a gym class. The phobic adolescent shows an irrational fear of school and may show marked anxiety symptoms when in or near the school.

---

**Useful instruments for screening for mental health problems in adolescents**

| Name of tool (inventor) | Scope of screening | No of items (time needed, minutes) |
|---|---|---|
| Beck depression inventory (Beck) | Depressive state | 21 (5) |
| SCL-90-R (Derogatis) | Mental health problems | 90 (12-15) |
| Brief symptom inventory (Derogatis) | Mental health problems | 53 (8-10) |
| Children's depression inventory (Kovacs) | Depression | 27 (5-10) |
| Strengths and difficulties questionnaire (Goodman) | General psychopathology and associated impairment | 25 or 30 (5-10) |
| Child behaviour checklist; youth self report (Achenbach) | General psychopathology | 120 (25) |
| Giessen test | Psychopathology | 30 (5-10) |

The brief symptom inventory is a shortened version of the SCL-90-R.

---

**Potential risk factors for adolescent depression**

- Family history of depression
- Recent bereavement or family conflict
- Break up of a romantic relationship
- Having a chronic medical condition
- Physical and sexual abuse
- Trauma and severe stress
- Anxiety, attention-deficit/hyperactivity disorder, or behavioural problems
- Learning difficulties
- Substance misuse

---

**Treatment strategies for adolescent depression**

**Brief psychological therapies**
- Cognitive behaviour therapy
- Interpersonal psychotherapy

**Longer term psychotherapy**
- Longer term psychodynamic therapies may be useful in more severe or persistent cases

**Antidepressants**
- Antidepressants are less effective in adolescents than in adults
- US and UK doctors have recently been warned that some selective serotonin reuptake inhibitors (SSRIs) may increase the risk of suicidal behaviour in adolescents. The only SSRI approved in the United Kingdom for adolescent depression is fluoxetine

---

**Cognitive behaviour therapy, usually for 12-16 weeks, is the treatment of choice for most adolescent depression; however, although cognitive behaviour therapy by general practitioners is effective in adults, its effectiveness is yet to be confirmed in adolescents**

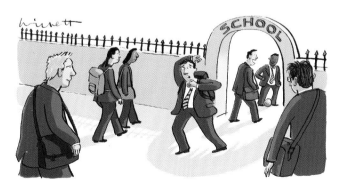

School phobia often occurs alongside social and other phobias and may be quite disabling, leading to failure in school and later vocational failure. Management usually requires involvement of the young person's whole "system"—including parents, siblings, and the school. Short term cognitive behaviour therapy, as well as selective serotonin reuptake inhibitors, has also been shown to be effective.

## Learning disabilities

Learning disability encompasses disorders that affect the way individuals with normal or above normal intelligence receive, store, organise, retrieve, and use information. Problems include dyslexia and other specific learning problems involving reading, spelling, writing, reasoning, and mathematics.

Undiagnosed learning disabilities are a common but manageable cause of young people deciding to leave school at the earliest opportunity. The clinicians' role in these situations is to screen for health conditions that may affect performance (such as hearing or vision problems or neurological disorders) and to identify psychosocial and environmental factors that may affect learning abilities (such as family disruption, poor peer relationships, or cultural and economic difficulties).

## Conduct disorders

Conduct disorder can be defined as persistently disruptive behaviour in which the young person repeatedly violates the rights of others or age appropriate social norms. It is often preceded by oppositionality and defiance in early years and can become more disruptive during adolescence. Symptoms include damage to property, lying or theft, truancy, violations of rules, and aggression towards people or animals. Teenagers with a conduct disorder often have concomitant disorders such as depression, suicidal behaviour, and poor relationships with peers and adults. Consequences include school problems, school expulsions, academic and vocational failure, and problems with the law. Parents and families need support to help them make sure that the young person does not stay away from school, and severely affected adolescents should be referred to mental health professionals for evaluation and care.

## Attention-deficit/hyperactivity disorder

Definitions of the symptom complex known as attention-deficit/hyperactivity disorder (ADHD) differ, but severe problems with concentration or attention and/or hyperactivity are estimated to affect about 5% of adolescents (Kondo et al, see "Further reading" box). Six times as many boys as girls are affected. The main consequences of ADHD are poor academic performance and behavioural problems, although adolescents with ADHD are at substantially higher risk of serious accidents, depression, and other psychological problems. About 80% of children with ADHD continue to have the disorder during adolescence, and as many as 50% of adolescents still do throughout adulthood. The main differential diagnoses are with behavioural problems secondary to poor parenting or poor school supervision.

Milder forms of ADHD can be amenable to simple management strategies. More severe problems may require treatment, including educational changes, behavioural programmes, family therapy, individual counselling, and the use of stimulant medications such as methylphenidate and dexamphetamine. Although the use of such stimulants remains

### Behaviour disorders

Behaviour disorders present difficulties for families, social services, and education

They rarely present as a clinical problem in primary or secondary care

Clinicians may become involved when there are other comorbid conditions (such as depression or substance misuse) and when other family members are affected by the young person's behaviour

Behaviour disorders rarely manifest for the first time in adolescence; the sudden development of new behaviour problems in adolescence may reflect underlying family problems, depression, or substance misuse

---

**Although severe learning problems present in early primary school, more subtle difficulties may be missed until made obvious by the greater academic demands of adolescence when they begin to affect educational performance**

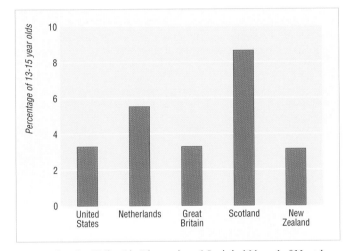

Conduct disorder (defined in Diagnostic and Statistical Manual of Mental Disorders, fourth edition) in 13-15 year olds in selected countries. Data from West et al (*J Am Acad Child Adolesc Psychiatry* 2003;42:941-9); Ford et al (*J Am Acad Child Adolesc Psychiatry* 2003;42:1203-11); Verhulst et al (*Arch Gen Psychiatry* 1997;54:329-36); Costello et al (*Arch Gen Psychiatry* 2003;60:837-44)

---

### Symptoms suggestive of attention-deficit/hyperactivity disorder (ADHD)*

**Inattention**
- Often fails to give close attention to details or makes careless mistakes in school work
- Often has difficulty sustaining attention in tasks or play activities
- Often does not seem to listen when spoken to directly
- Often does not follow through on instructions and fails to finish school work, chores, duties in the workplace
- Often has difficulty organising tasks and activities
- Often is distracted by extranaeous stimuli and is forgetful in daily activities

**Hyperactivity**
- Often fidgets with hands or feet or squirms in seat
- Often leaves seat in classroom or other situation where it is inappropriate (or, more usually in adolescents, just feelings of restlessness)
- Often runs about or climbs excessively in situations where this is inappropriate (or, more usually in adolescents, just feelings of restlessness)

*Kondo et al (see "Further Reading" box)

controversial, there is strong evidence that they improve educational and behavioural outcomes. However, they should be prescribed only in secondary care and only after a full psychiatric and medical investigation.

# Anxiety disorders

Anxiety disorders are relatively common in adolescents and often persist into adulthood. Whereas separation anxiety disorder and mutism are more prevalent among younger children, generalised anxiety disorder and panic attacks emerge during adolescence. Generalised anxiety disorder is marked by uncontrolled excessive worrying, accompanied by difficulty in concentrating, irritability, sleep problems, and often fatigue. Panic disorder is characterised by recurrent spontaneous panic attacks, often associated with physiological and psychological signs and symptoms. As with other mental health problems in adolescence, anxiety disorders are often accompanied by other conditions, particularly depression.

As many anxiety disorders during adolescence are accompanied by physical symptoms, careful evaluation is needed—at least a complete medical history and a comprehensive physical examination—to exclude conditions such as hypoglycaemic episodes, migraine, seizure, and other neurological problems. Treatment may include simple educational strategies, behavioural interventions, cognitive behaviour therapy, family therapy, and rarely, the use of anxiolytics.

The photograph is reproduced with permission from Robin M White/ Photonica.

---

**Behavioural strategies for attention-deficit/hyperactivity disorder (ADHD)***

*At home (parents)*—Use simple commands; set defined limits and expectations; praise and reinforce desired behaviours (rewards); establish a formal structure for time schedules; use lists and calendars to help prevent forgetfulness; break long tasks into shorter ones

*At school (teachers)*—Ensure that the young person sits close to the teacher's desk (away from distractions); give only one task at a time (with assignments as short as possible); use written not just oral instructions for homework (in notebook to be taken home); do a daily or weekly report; allow more time for examinations (including untimed tests); ensure than young person can rely on a neighbouring student; ask for the help of a trained specialist tutor

*Kondo et al (see "Further Reading" box)

---

**General practitioners must take a substantial role in detecting and treating such problems in order to reduce the overall burden of adolescent mental health problems on individuals and society**

---

**Further reading**

- World Health Organization. *Invest in mental health.* Geneva: WHO, 2003.
- Rutter M, Smith D. *Psychosocial disorders in young people. Time trends and their causes.* New York: Wiley, 1995.
- Meltzer H, Gatward R, Goodam R, Ford T. *The mental health of children and adolescents in Great Britain.* 2nd ed. London: Office for National Statistics, 2000.
- Bower P, Garralda E, Kramer T, Harrington R, Sibbald B. The treatment of child and adolescent mental health problems in primary care: a systematic review. *Fam Pract* 2001;18:373-82.
- Hack S, Jellinek M. Early identification of emotional and behavioral problems in a primary care setting. In: Juszczak LFM, ed. *Adolescent medicine: state of the art reviews.* Philadelphia: Belfus Ha, 1996:335-50.
- Michael KD, Crowley SL. How effective are treatments for child and adolescent depression? A meta-analytic review. *Clin Psychol Rev* 2002;22:247-69.
- Kondo DG, Chrisman AK, March JS. An evidence-based medicine approach to combined treatment for ADHD in children and adolescents. *Psychopharmacol Bull* 2003;37(3):7-23.

# 10   Suicide and deliberate self harm in young people

Keith Hawton, Anthony James

Deliberate self harm ranges from behaviours with no suicidal intent (but with the intent to communicate distress or relieve tension) through to suicide. Some 7%-14% of adolescents will self harm at some time in their life, and 20%-45% of older adolescents report having had suicidal thoughts at some time.

## Suicide

Suicide occurs relatively rarely under the age of 15 years, although prevalence is likely to be underestimated because of reluctance of coroners to assign this verdict. A large proportion of open verdicts ("undetermined cause") are, in fact, suicides. Suicide rates are far higher in male than female adolescents. Until the past five or six years in England and Wales suicide rates were rising substantially in 15-19 year old and 20-24 year old young men, but then they began to fall somewhat in the older age group. The lack of change in female suicide rates may reflect differential effects of social change on gender roles.

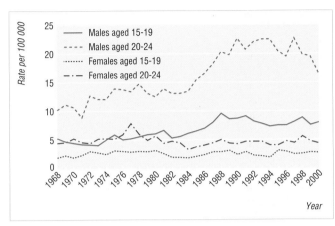

Suicide and undetermined deaths in England and Wales in 15-19 year olds and 20-24 year olds between 1968 and 2000. Data source: Office for National Statistics. *Twentieth century mortality: 100 years of mortality data in England and Wales by age, sex, year and underlying cause.* CD Rom. London: ONS, 2003.

---

**Possible reasons for rise in male suicide rates in United Kingdom**

- Increased rates of family breakdown
- Increasing rates of substance misuse
- Increasing rates of depression
- Greater instability of employment
- Increased availability of means for suicide
- Media influences (thought to contribute to 5% of suicides in adolescents)
- Awareness of suicidal behaviour in other young people

---

Psychological postmortem studies of suicides show that a psychiatric disorder (usually depression, rarely psychosis) is present at the time of death in most adolescents who die by suicide. A history of behavioural disturbance, substance misuse, and family, social, and psychological problems is common. There are strong links between suicide and previous self harm: between a quarter and a half of those committing suicide have previously carried out a non-fatal act.

## Deliberate self harm

The term deliberate self harm is preferred to "attempted suicide" or "parasuicide" because the range of motives or reasons for this behaviour includes several non-suicidal intentions. Although adolescents who self harm may claim they want to die, the motivation in many is more to do with an expression of distress and desire for escape from troubling situations. Even when death is the outcome of self harming behaviour, this may not have been intended.

Most self harm in adolescents inflicts little actual harm and does not come to the attention of medical services. Self cutting is involved in many such cases and appears to serve the purpose of reducing tension or of self punishment. By contrast, self poisoning makes up about 90% of cases referred to hospital. The substances involved are usually readily available in the home or can be bought over the counter and include non-opiate analgesics—such as paracetamol and aspirin—and

---

**Common characteristics of adolescents who die by suicide**

- Broken homes (separation, divorce, or death of parents)
- Family psychiatric disorder or suicidal behaviour
- Psychiatric disorder or behavioural disturbance
- Substance misuse (alcohol or drugs)
- Previous self harm

---

**Common expressions of parental grief after suicide by adolescents**

- Refusal to accept that the death was a suicide
- Anger towards friends of the deceased, family members, medical staff, coroners, and even the deceased person
- Guilt
- Shame
- Constant search for explanation
- Fear of welfare of other children; overprotection
- Disruption of relationship with partner
- Stigmatisation
- Depression or suicidal ideation
- Alcohol misuse

---

**General practitioners, bereavement counsellors, support organisations, and the clergy have important roles in providing support and facilitating grief**

---

**Possible motives or reasons underlying self harm**
- To die
- To escape from unbearable anguish
- To change the behaviour of others
- To escape from a situation
- To show desperation to others
- To change the behaviour of others
- To "get back at" other people or make them feel guilty
- To gain relief of tension
- To seek help

---

psychotropic agents. Self harm by more dangerous methods, such as attempted hanging, may be associated with considerable suicidal intent.

### Risk factors

Common characteristics of adolescents who self harm are similar to the characteristics of those who commit suicide. Physical or sexual abuse may also be a factor. Recently there has been increasing recognition of the importance of depression in non-fatal as well as fatal self harm by adolescents. Substance misuse is also common, although the degree of risk of self harm in adolescents attributable to alcohol or drug misuse is unclear. Knowing others who self harm may be an important factor.

Young South Asian females in the United Kingdom seem to have a raised risk of self harm. Intercultural stresses and consequent family conflicts may be relevant factors.

As many as 30% of adolescents who self harm report previous episodes, many of which have not come to medical attention. At least 10% repeat self harm during the following year, with repeats being especially likely in the first two or three months.

The risk of suicide after deliberate self harm varies between 0.24% and 4.30%. Our knowledge of risk factors is limited and can be used only as an adjunct to careful clinical assessment when making decisions about after care. However, the following factors seem to indicate a risk: being an older teenage male; violent method of self harm; multiple previous episodes of self harm; apathy, hopelessness, and insomnia; substance misuse; and previous admission to a psychiatric hospital.

## Prevention

It can be difficult to identify young people at risk of self harm, even though many older adolescents who are at risk consult their general practitioners before they self harm. Suicidal ideation is relatively common among adolescents; precipitating events may be non-specific; acts of self harm are often impulsive; and secrecy and denial are common. Effective preventive care requires involvement of multiple agencies—for example, mental health services and social services. These agencies need to work in a coordinated way with adolescents thought to be at risk, including those with severe psychiatric disorders.

## Assessment after self harm

All young people who have self harmed in a potentially serious way should be assessed in hospital by either a child and adolescent psychiatrist or a specialist mental health worker, psychologist, psychotherapist, or psychiatric nurse. This is necessary for the management of the medical issues and to ensure the young person receives a thorough psychosocial assessment.

The clinician can improve his or her examination by using a semistructured assessment. The natural starting point is inquiry about the events leading up to the act.

It is essential to establish whether the young person had a high degree of suicidal intent. As denial of intent is sometimes a problem, it is important to get as detailed an account of the circumstances as possible and compare these to factors known to be associated with high intent. Sometimes the reasons for self harm seen unclear because the act may seem highly impulsive. The clinician must therefore use all the information available to try to understand the motivation. This should involve exploring the adolescent's concept of death—asking, for example, what they expected to happen and whether they had thought they

**Self harm is frequently a highly impulsive act—many individuals report that they had thought about the act for just minutes before doing it. Alcohol and drug consumption probably increases the likelihood of impulsive acts**

---

### Common problems preceding self harm

- Difficulties or disputes with parents
- School or work problems
- Difficulties with boyfriends or girlfriends
- Disputes with siblings
- Physical ill health
- Difficulties or disputes with peers
- Depression
- Bullying
- Low self esteem
- Sexual problems
- Alcohol and drug abuse
- Awareness of self harm by friends or family

---

### Factors associated with repeated self harm

- Previous self harm
- Personality disturbance
- Depression
- Alcohol or drug misuse
- Chronic psychosocial problems and behaviour disturbance
- Disturbed family relationships
- Alcohol dependence in the family
- Social isolation
- Poor school record

---

### Groups at risk who may benefit from preventive strategies

- Depressed adolescents (depression may be less easy to identify in adolescents than in adults because of atypical presentation, such as behavioural disturbance, poor school performance, and social withdrawal)
- Those with an interpersonal crisis, such as loss of a partner or running away from home
- Those who have previously self harmed, particularly if substance misuse and conduct disorder are present

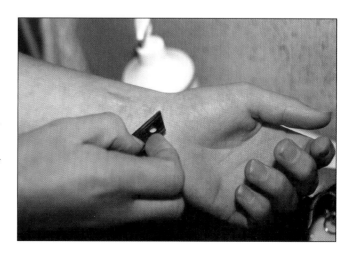

would still be around afterwards to see the consequences of the act. Suicidal intent tends to be associated with depression and hopelessness.

The physical severity of the self harm is not a good indicator of suicidal intent because adolescents are often unaware of the relative toxicity of supposedly harmless substances such as paracetamol. Similar issues in the young person and their family can be usefully assessed in primary care in cases of less serious self harm.

## Features of self harm that suggest high suicidal intent

- Conducted in isolation
- Timed so that intervention is unlikely (for example, after parents have gone to work)
- Precautions to avoid discovery
- Preparations made in anticipation of death (for example, leaving indication of how belongings to be distributed)
- Adolescent told other people beforehand about thoughts of suicide
- The act had been considered for hours or days beforehand
- Suicide note or message
- Adolescent did not alert others during or after the act

# Treatment

Most adolescents who self harm do so in response to interpersonal crises and can be discharged for treatment as outpatients. Inpatient psychiatric treatment is usually reserved for those who have severe depressive or psychotic disorder, present an ongoing risk of suicide, or are in the middle of major psychosocial difficulties, such as disclosure of sexual abuse.

A crisis intervention model is often most appropriate. Compliance, however, can be a problem because the self harm may have had a positive effect by providing temporary relief from a difficult situation. Also the take-up of treatment depends largely on parental background and attitudes, which may include denial and negative views about psychological help. A home based treatment programme may overcome some of these problems.

Problem solving therapy is often used with adolescents and has the advantage of being direct and easily understood. Using problem solving techniques and rehearsing coping strategies can help the adolescent when he or she is confronted with future crises.

The problem solving approach can also be extended to involve the whole family. Family interventions are structured, usually last five or six sessions, and can be home based. Essential elements include the improvement of specific cognitive and social skills to promote the sharing of feelings, emotional control, and negotiation between family members. Role play can be a useful additional technique. It is wise to anticipate crises by making provision for appointments at short notice or giving telephone numbers for emergencies. Adolescents who self harm can also be treated in groups.

If depression is present, cognitive behaviour therapy is an effective treatment in adolescents. The selective serotonin reuptake inhibitor fluoxetine (Prozac) is effective in this age group. However, in view of the risk of further self harm by overdose, it is wise to limit supplies of this drug and get other family members to handle it, at least initially.

If school problems, particularly bullying, are prominent, liaison with the school is important. Further help may be provided by a school counsellor. In the case of learning difficulties, an assessment by an educational psychologist may be helpful in devising suitable educational options.

## Important issues in assessment of adolescents who have self harmed

- Events surrounding the overdose or self harm
- Degree of suicidal intent and other reasons for the act
- The adolescent's current problems
- Possible psychiatric disorder
- Family and personal history
- History of psychiatric disorder or self harm
- The nature of the adolescent's resources and supports
- Risk of further self harm and of suicide
- Attitudes towards help

## Assessment of families of young people who seriously self harm

### Elements of assessment
- Family structure and relationships
- History of psychiatric disorder, including suicide attempts in the family
- Recent family life events, especially losses

### Assessment of family's support and problem solving ability
- Inquire about the circumstances of the self harm, events leading up to it, and how it has affected the family
- Inquire about how the family has tackled serious problems in the past

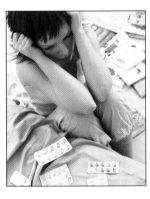

Self poisoning is the second most common method (after self cutting) for deliberate self harm by adolescents

## Treatment options for adolescent self harm

### Individual
- Problem solving
- Cognitive behavioural therapy
- Treatment of underlying psychiatric disorder (such as antidepressants or cognitive behaviour therapy)
- Treatment of drug or alcohol abuse
- Anger management

### Family
- Family therapy (such as problem solving or structural or systemic therapy)

### Group
- Group therapy (including problem solving, cognitive behavioural therapy, and dealing with developmental concerns and emotions)

### Others
- Environmental changes (such as temporary alternative accommodation)

## Basics of problem solving therapy

- Identifying and deciding what problem(s) to tackle first
- Agreeing goals
- Working out steps to achieve goals
- Deciding how to tackle the first step
- Reviewing progress
- Dealing with psychological factors that obstruct progress
- Working through subsequent steps

When the self harm occurs alongside substance and alcohol misuse or violence, specific treatments for these conditions may be indicated. For older adolescents, referral to a self help agency or walk-in counselling service may be appropriate—and more readily accepted.

## Further reading

- Fox C, Hawton K. *Deliberate self harm in adolescence.* London: Jessica Kingsley, 2004.
- Gould M, Greenberg T, Velting DM, Shaffer D. Youth suicide risk and preventive interventions: a review of the past ten years. *J Am Acad Child Adolesc Psychiatry* 2003;42:386-405.
- Hawton K, Hall S, Simkin S, Bale L, Bond A, Codd S, et al. Deliberate self-harm in adolescents: a study of characteristics and trends in Oxford, 1999-2000. *J Child Psychol Psychiatry* 2003;44:1191-8.
- Hawton K, Rodham K, Evans E, Weatherall R. Deliberate self-harm in adolescents: self report survey in schools in England. *BMJ* 2002;325:1207-11.
- Wood A, Trainor G, Rothwell J, Moore A, Harrington R. Randomized trial of group therapy for repeated deliberate self-harm in adolescents. *J Am Acad Child Adolesc Psychiatry* 2001;40:1246-53.

## Information resources

### For young people

- *Depression in children and young people.* Factsheet 21. From Royal College of Psychiatrists (RCPsych), tel 020 7235 2351; www.rcpsych.ac.uk

### For parents and teachers

- *Suicide and self-harm in people.* Factsheet 15. From RCPsych (as above).
- Graham P, Hughes C. *So young, so sad, so listen.* London: Gaskell, 1995.
- www.youngminds.org.uk (YoungMinds is a national charity working to improve the mental health of all children and young people).
- www.euteach.com (for information on teaching about mental health issues in young people).

### For parents and others bereaved by suicide

- Hill K, Hawton K, Malmberg A, Simkin S. *Bereavement information pack: for those bereaved by suicide or other sudden death.* London: Gaskell, 1997. Available via RCPsych (as above) and at www.rcpsych.ac.uk/publications/gaskell/bereav/index.htm
- Wertheimer A. *A special scar: the experiences of people bereaved by suicide.* 2nd ed. London: Brunner-Routledge, 2001.

The two photographs are reproduced with permission from Tor Richard Simonsen/Rex (self cutting) and BSIP.Chassenet/SPL (self poisoning).

# 11   Eating disorders and weight problems

Dasha Nicholls, Russell Viner

Adolescence is a time of enormous change in weight and eating. Average weight gain during puberty is 14 kg for girls and 15 kg for boys, with marked differences in body shape between the sexes becoming evident. About 40% of girls (25% of boys) begin dieting in adolescence. Reported dieting may often reflect dissatisfaction with their body rather than actual calorie restriction. Six to 12 per cent of adolescents choose to become vegetarian, giving them increased independence from family eating patterns.

Eating disorders, anorexia nervosa, and bulimia nervosa, are characterised by morbid preoccupation with weight and shape and manifest through distorted or chaotic eating behaviour. This behaviour differentiates these disorders from other types of psychological problems associated with abnormal eating behaviour—such as extreme faddy (selective) eating and various types of food phobia—and from obesity, in which primary psychological mechanisms are rarely implicated or are part of a more complex picture.

## Eating disorders

Studies have found anorexia nervosa to be the third commonest chronic illness of adolescence, affecting 0.5% of adolescent girls. Bulimia nervosa is slightly more common (1%), but the secretive nature of the disorder and adolescents' reluctance to seek help mean that it is often hidden.

Eating disorders occur in all ethnic groups, and about 90% of cases are in females. Social, psychological (perception of ideal body weight and individual temperament), and genetic mechanisms all contribute to the development of an eating disorder.

### Recognition

The diagnosis of eating disorders in adolescents should take into consideration the context of normal pubertal growth and adolescent development. Although the problem may present as a result of other people's concern, assessment of the young person on their own is necessary to establish diagnosis, risk, and attitude to help. Diagnostic criteria are helpful, but intervention should also be considered in adolescents with severely abnormal eating attitudes and behaviours (such as those who vomit or take laxatives regularly but do not binge) or whose rate of weight loss is of more concern than degree of underweight.

**For some young people, eating behaviours such as dieting that develop during adolescence can herald the onset of more serious eating problems**

---

**Prevalence of eating behaviours and eating problems in adolescence in United Kingdom**

| Eating behaviour | Prevalence (%) | Sex ratio (female to male) |
|---|---|---|
| Dieting | 35 | 1.5:1 |
| Anorexia nervosa | 0.4 | 9:1 |
| Bulimia nervosa | 1 | 30:1 |
| Obesity | 7-10 | 1.3:1 |

---

**Risk factors for developing eating disorder in adolescence**

- Female sex
- Repeated dieting
- Early puberty
- Temperament
- Perfectionism
- Teasing about weight and dieting
- Low self esteem
- Losses and major life events
- Family dysfunction

---

**Differentiation of anorexia from bulimia**

| Anorexia nervosa | Bulimia nervosa |
|---|---|
| Low weight | Normal weight |
| Presents early | Presents late |
| Patient rarely seeks help | Patient may seek help |
| Onset early to middle teens | Onset late teens |
| Can be premenarcheal | Is rarely premenarcheal |
| Can affect boys | Usually affects girls |
| Acute or chronic | Fluctuating course |
| No previous illness | Previous anorexia nervosa |
| Associated with anxiety, obsessive compulsive disorder, depression | Associated with depression, self harm, substance misuse |
| Prognosis poor without early intervention | Up to 60% respond to specific treatments |

---

**Diagnostic criteria for anorexia nervosa and bulimia nervosa\***

**Anorexia nervosa**
- Body weight is maintained at least 15% below that expected or body mass index is 17.5 or lower†
- Weight loss is self induced by avoidance of "fattening foods" plus one or more of: self induced vomiting; self induced purging; excessive exercise; use of appetite suppressants or diuretics
- Body image distortion in which dread of fatness persists as an intrusive, overvalued idea
- Widespread endocrine disorder involving the hypothalamic-pituitary-gonadal and manifesting as amenorrhoea in women and loss of sexual interest and potency in men
- If onset is prepubertal, puberty is delayed or arrested. With recovery, puberty is often normal, but the menarche is late

**Bulimia nervosa**
- Persistent preoccupation with eating; overeating episodes in which large amounts of food are eaten in short periods of time
- The patient tries to counteract the "fattening" effects of food by one or more of: self induced vomiting or purgative abuse; alternating starvation and eating; use of appetite suppressants, thyroid preparations, or diuretics
- The psychopathology consists of a morbid dread of fatness, and the patient sets herself or himself a precise weight threshold, well below the premorbid weight that constitutes the optimum or healthy weight in the opinion of the physician
- Often a history of previous anorexia nervosa, with the interval ranging from a few months to several years

\*Based on ICD-10 (international classification of diseases, 10th revision); †Body mass index criterion does not apply for young people aged under 17

The body mass index (BMI (kg/m²)) is misleading in children and adolescents, and BMI centiles must be used to define underweight. A BMI lower than the ≤2nd centile indicates serious underweight and should be a trigger for referral. An eating disorder should also be considered if an adolescent fails to attain or maintain a healthy weight, height, or stage of sexual maturity for age.

Once the patient has been weighed and their height measured, a few key questions (how much would you like to weigh? how do you feel about your weight? are you or is anyone else worried about your eating or exercising?)—asked in a non-judgmental manner—can be helpful in deciding whether further assessment is needed. An adolescent's distress about being asked about weight and food should heighten concern. If the concern is equivocal, a further appointment within a month is advisable.

## Psychological or behavioural markers of potential eating disorder

- Is a reluctant attender at the surgery or clinic
- Seeks help for physical symptoms
- Resists weighing and examination
- Covers body
- Is secretive or evasive
- Has increased energy (and in some cases agitation)
- Gets angry or distressed when asked about eating problems

**Physical signs of malnutrition and purging include thinning hair, parotid gland swelling, enamel erosion, hypothermia, bradycardia, lanugo hair, dry skin, hypotension, underweight, cold hands and blue/mottled peripheries, poor capillary return, carotenaemia, insensitivity to pain, constipation, amenorrhoea, shrunken breasts**

After an eating disorder is identified, direct challenge or confrontation is unlikely to be helpful. At first presentation aim to (a) feed back findings from physical examination, including degree of underweight if relevant; (b) establish weight monitoring plus a plan to follow if weight falls; (c) discuss psychiatric risk as needed; and (d) provide the family and young person with information about the nature, course, and treatment of eating disorders. In general, the threshold for intervention should be lower for adolescents than for adults.

## Management

Assessment and management of a young person with an identified eating disorder needs to tackle medical, nutritional, and psychological aspects of care and be delivered by healthcare staff who are knowledgeable about normal adolescent development. When management is shared between primary and secondary care, clear agreement is needed about who is responsible for monitoring patients, and this should be communicated to the patient and his or her family.

Management of nutritional disturbances in adolescents with eating disorders should take into account the pubertal development and activity level. This is likely to mean that they will need a higher calorie intake for adequate weight gain than the intake required by adult patients with eating disorders.

Family interventions that directly tackle the eating disorder should be offered to adolescents with anorexia nervosa. Adolescents with bulimia nervosa may best be treated with cognitive behaviour therapy specific to the disorder, with the family included as appropriate. Consideration should be given

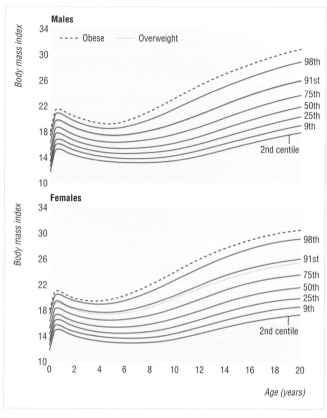

Body mass index charts (showing centiles and BMI values for overweight and obesity at age 18) for assessing underweight; the trigger for referring a young person with serious underweight to a specialist is a body mass index lower than or equal to the second centile

**For young people under 16 years who present alone with an eating disorder, communication with parents or carers will need to be discussed**

## Criteria for considering admission to hospital for anorexia nervosa

- Very rapid weight loss or very low energy intake
- Body mass index substantially below the second centile
- High risk of suicide
- Signs of physical compromise (severe dehydration; capillary return ≥1.5 seconds; resting pulse ≤45 beats/min; diastolic blood pressure ≤40 mm Hg and/or very wide pulse pressure or severe postural hypotension)

## Consequences of eating disorders

### Short term
- Sinus bradycardia; T wave inversions; ST segment depression; prolonged corrected QT interval; dysrhythmias with supraventricular beats and ventricular tachycardia
- Slowed gastrointestinal motility and constipation; abnormal results on liver function tests; superior mesenteric artery syndrome
- Raised blood urea nitrogen concentration with increased risk of renal stones
- Leucopenia; anaemia; iron deficiency; thrombocytopenia
- Sick euthyroid syndrome; amenorrhoea

### Long term
- Pubertal delay or arrest
- Growth retardation and short stature
- Impairment of bone mineral acquisition, leading to osteopenia or osteoporosis
- Psychological sequelae—for example, anxiety and depression

to the impact of the problem on siblings, who should be involved in treatment when possible.

Admission to hospital is necessary if there is acute physical compromise, high psychiatric risk, or after an adequate trial of outpatient treatment. Admission may be to a paediatric ward, an adolescent psychiatric unit, or a specialist eating disorders unit. These facilities should provide skilled feeding with careful physical monitoring (particularly in the first few days) together with psychosocial interventions.

# Obesity

Rates of obesity have increased substantially among children and adolescents in almost all developed countries in the past two decades. In the United Kingdom, an estimated 7-8% of adolescents of both sexes are seriously obese, with a further 15% being seriously overweight but not obese. The great majority of child and adolescent obesity is primary in origin, due to a long term imbalance between nutritional intake and energy expenditure. Identified monogenic syndromes and secondary causes of obesity probably account for less than 1% of adolescent obesity.

Obesity in adolescence is a concern because it is associated with current as well as future health problems. Type 2 diabetes and the insulin resistance (metabolic) syndrome are emerging as problems in adolescence. Clinical data suggest that as many as 4% of obese adolescents may have silent type 2 diabetes and a further 30% may have three or more components of the insulin resistance syndrome.

## Assessment

The most useful definition of obesity is that developed by the International Obesity Task Force, which found that the BMI 99th centile approximately equates to 30 (which in adults is the level linked with adverse health outcomes). As highly muscular young people can have a high BMI yet a low fat mass, it is best to also use a second method of assessing body fat mass, such as waist circumference (for which centiles are now available) or bioimpedance measure (centiles being developed). Those with both a high BMI and a high waist circumference are probably at highest risk.

### Medical assessment

Family history of obesity and the family risk profile in terms of history of diabetes and components of the insulin resistance syndrome should be noted. Ethnic background should also be considered, as those from a black or South Asian background have a significantly higher risk of the insulin resistance syndrome and diabetes.

On clinical examination, important signs include fat distribution (generalised or abdominal), acanthosis nigricans (a marker of hyperinsulinism), pubertal development, and blood pressure (measured with an appropriate size cuff). In girls, hirsuitism and acne may suggest polycystic ovarian syndrome. It is useful to search for signs of hypothyroidism and Cushing's syndrome, although obesity is rarely the sole presentation of these conditions in adolescence. Striae and a prominent nuchal fat pad ("buffalo hump") are extremely common in adolescents with simple obesity.

Minimal investigations should be done in primary care in adolescents thought to be at high risk (high BMI, abdominal obesity, family history of diabetes or of the insulin resistance syndrome). These include simple biochemistry and haematology tests, fasting insulin and glucose tests, fasting lipid tests, and thyroid function tests.

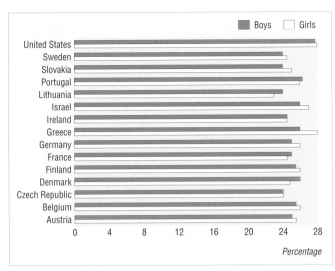

Percentage of 15 year olds who are obese in Europe and the United States. Adapted from Lissau et al. *Arch Pediatr Adolesc Med* 2004;158:27-33

---

**Conditions associated with obesity**

**Current**
- Type 2 diabetes
- Insulin resistance (metabolic) syndrome: hyperinsulinism, dyslipidaemia, hypertension
- Polycystic ovarian syndrome
- Non-alcoholic steatohepatitis
- Asthma
- Psychological morbidity, including higher rates of low self esteem, depression, suicide attempts
- Poor academic achievement
- Arthritis

**Future**
- Excess mortality (from cardiovascular disease, cancer, all causes)
- Reduced professional, financial, and marital expectations

---

**Aims of obesity assessment**

- To categorise cardiovascular risk profile (elements of the insulin resistance syndrome: fasting hyperinsulinaemia; hypertension; dyslipidaemia; obesity, particularly abdominal obesity; type 2 diabetes)
- To identify current or potential complications of obesity
- To exclude secondary causes of obesity: genetic causes (such as Prader-Willi syndrome, Bardet Biedl syndrome, and rare monogenic syndromes) and endocrine syndromes such as hypothyroidism and Cushing's syndrome

---

**Important issues in taking a history in adolescent obesity**

**Plotting the "obesity trajectory"**
To do this we ask about birth weight; about early feeding history; whether onset of obesity was sudden or gradual, and at what age; whether progression of obesity was rapid or gradual; whether there have been any periods of very rapid weight gain, particularly recently; whether there have been any periods of weight loss (and why and how achieved); who else in the family is obese or has trouble controlling their weight

**Family risk profile**
To place the child in the appropriate risk category ask about family history of components of the insulin resistance syndrome (morbid obesity; type 2 diabetes; hypertension; dyslipidaemia; polycystic ovarian syndrome; early cardiovascular disease (defined as development of cardiovascular disease at age 50-59 or younger)

## Treatment

The treatment of obesity is notoriously difficult, and a lack of belief that obesity can be treated is widespread. In the United Kingdom, the Royal College of Paediatrics and Child Health has recently issued excellent brief guidance on managing obesity in primary care.

The most successful obesity treatments are multidisciplinary programmes that urge changes in eating habits and family systems and promote exercise and a reduction in sedentary activities. Dietary interventions alone are unlikely to produce substantial change.

A treatment plan should be guided by an assessment of risk in both the medical and psychological domains. The psychological domains include emotional overeating, substantial distress, parental mental health, and (rarely) child protection concerns. Substantial weight loss is extremely difficult to achieve, and setting overambitious targets can reduce motivation. Our primary aim in adolescents who are still growing is weight maintenance, thereby producing loss of overweight. As this is achievable only before the end of the pubertal growth spurt, obesity should be treated before puberty if possible. Secondary aims may include improvement in psychological wellbeing; family functioning; and insulin sensitivity, liver function, and lipid concentrations.

The limited effectiveness of treatment has prompted a reconsideration of the role of drugs in severe obesity. No drugs for the treatment of obesity in childhood are currently approved in the United Kingdom or the United States. Metformin, orlistat, and sibutramine may be used in specialist centres. Drug treatment is more effective when combined with a behavioural intervention.

The most effective ways to prevent and treat obesity are likely to be actions at the macroeconomic level. However, in local communities, individual clinicians may be able to encourage change by promoting simple measures to allow adolescents to participate in sport and activity and eat more healthily.

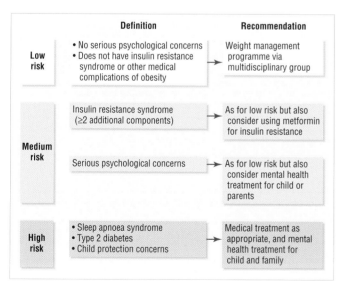

Assessment of risk and treatment options

### Guidelines for treatment of obesity in primary care*

**Features that should trigger referral to paediatrician**
- Serious morbidity related to obesity (such as sleep apnoea, orthopaedic problems, type 2 and non-insulin dependent diabetes mellitus, hypertension)
- Height below 9th centile, unexpectedly short for family, or slowed growth rate
- Precocious or late puberty (before 8 years, or no signs at 13 in girls or 15 in boys)
- Severe learning disability
- Symptoms and signs of genetic or endocrine abnormalities
- Severe and progressive obesity before age 2
- Other serious concerns

**Weight management options and contraindications**
- No weight gain as height increases
- Weight gain slower than height gain
- Rapid weight loss and strict dieting are not appropriate for growing children unless under specialist care

**Action**
- Successful interventions involve the family and are tailored to each individual
- The multidisciplinary team needed may include a general practitioner, practice nurse, health visitor, school nurse, and other professionals if available (such as paediatric dietician, clinical psychologist, community paediatrician)
- Negotiate realistic goals and monitoring plans
- Provide information on local physical activity facilities, healthy eating, local parenting support groups

*Adapted from the Royal College of Paediatrics and Child Health and National Obesity Forum. *An Approach to Weight Management in Children and Adolescents (2-18 years) in Primary Care.* 2002 (www.rcpch.ac.uk/)

### Evidence for prevention of child and adolescent obesity

| Evidence for prevention | Longitudinal studies into adulthood | Longitudinal studies within childhood | Cross sectional studies in childhood |
|---|---|---|---|
| Sedentary activities | Yes | Yes | Yes |
| Exercise | Yes | Yes | Yes |
| Diet | No | No | Yes |
| Eating pattern (breakfast, family) | No | No | Yes |
| Breastfed as infant | Yes | Yes | Yes |

### Further reading and resources

- Mulvihill C, Quigley R. *Review of prevention of obesity. The management of obesity and overweight: an analysis of reviews of diet, physical activity and behavioural approaches.* London: Health Development Agency, 2003. (Evidence briefing.) (www.hda.nhs.uk/evidence)
- Campbell K, Waters E, O'Meara S, Kelly S, Summerbell CD. Interventions for preventing obesity in children. *Cochrane Database Syst Rev* 2004;(2):CD001871
- Gowers S, Bryant-Waugh R. The management of children and adolescents with eating disorders. *J Child Psychol Psychiatry* 2004;45:63-83
- Child Growth Foundation, 2 Mayfield Avenue, London W4 1PW and Harlow Printing, Maxwell Street, South Shields NE33 4PU UK (for BMI centile charts based on the UK 1990 growth reference and waist centile charts)
- www.nice.org.uk (for guidelines on eating disorders from the National Institute for Clinical Evidence)

# 12 Fatigue and somatic symptoms

Russell Viner, Deborah Christie

Fatigue, headache, stomach ache, and backache are common. Large international surveys show that about 8% of adolescents report daily headaches, 10% daily backache, and 16% daily sleepiness in the mornings. Fatigue is even more common—about a third of both boys and girls have substantial fatigue four or more times a week.

## Competing demands in adolescence

Most adolescents with these symptoms do not seek help from their doctor. They can present diagnostic dilemmas when they do, however. In most cases, the symptoms reflect not an organic disorder but an imbalance between the increasing educational, social, and sports demands on young people and physiological "debts" owed to rapid growth and sexual development. Adolescents, for example, need more sleep than children and adults, yet social and educational demands often mean that they sleep less. Adolescents may also have a physical hypersensitivity to changes in the growing body. For a minority, these symptoms may represent a functional or somatoform disorder, where psychological problems are expressed through physical symptoms rather than through language. Unexplained abdominal pain is a common example of this in early adolescents, with older adolescents more likely to have headaches or fatigue.

## Somatic symptoms

Signs or symptoms suggestive of more serious somatoform disorder include the co-occurrence of multiple symptoms (such as headaches with fatigue and muscle aches), chronicity (symptoms lasting more than three months), diminishing school attendance, and social isolation, together with a history of recent family, school, or psychological problems.

When pain or symptoms remain unexplained, they should be investigated with caution. Although it is important not to miss an organic disorder—and there is frequently family pressure to find an "answer"—repeated investigations can reduce the effectiveness of rehabilitation and symptom control.

After exclusion of common organic disorders, consider how the symptom affects the young person's school, social, and family life, as well as how much distress or pain the symptom causes. Take an adequate history—including social, school, and family issues—and assess whether bullying, depression, or family conflict may be contributing.

### Headaches

Headaches, along with stomach ache and backache, are the commonest chronic symptoms in adolescence apart from fatigue. The differential diagnosis can be fairly extensive. Most cases will be forms of muscular tension headaches. Migraine affects only about 2% of adolescents.

Other common causes of headache include extracranial problems (ear, sinus, or tooth infections, or temporomandibular joint disease) and excess caffeine consumption (from coffee or fizzy drinks). It is worth while excluding poor visual acuity as a cause of tension headaches. Uncommon causes of headaches

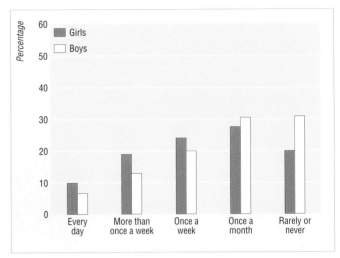

Frequency of headache in the previous six months in 11-17 year olds in Europe. Adapted from: World Health Organization. *Health behaviour in school-aged children, 1997-1998.* Calverton, MD: Macro International, 2002

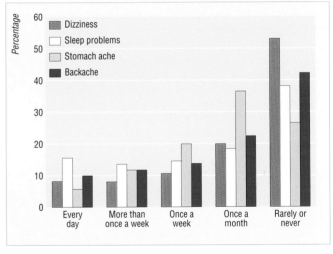

Prevalence of somatic symptoms (other than headache) in the previous six months in 11-17 year olds in Europe. Adapted from *Health behaviour in school-aged children, 1997-1998* (see above)

**Assess the young person's mood—symptoms associated with depressed mood (flat or constrained affect, being tearful, feeling hopeless, and loss of interest in friends and school), substantial loss of quality of life, or failure to attend school should be viewed with concern**

**Signs that further neurological evaluation of headaches is needed**

- Abrupt onset of, or sudden change in, symptoms
- Vomiting
- Morning headaches
- Headache wakes patient from sleep
- Reduction in school performance
- Associated seizures or neurological signs

are similar to those in adults, although it is important to note that benign intracranial hypertension is relatively more common in adolescence.

### Abdominal pain

Recurrent abdominal pain may present a particular diagnostic dilemma in early adolescents. This is particularly so in girls, in whom gynaecological causes of pain could be present. In older adolescents, the range of symptoms is more similar to that in adults. Upper abdominal pain may suggest non-ulcer dyspepsia, and *Helicobater pylori* infection should be excluded. Changes in bowel habit (such as diarrhoea or increased frequency of stools with pain that is relieved by defecation) may suggest irritable bowel syndrome, which can be seen from mid-adolescence onwards.

## Fatigue

Fatigue is almost a "normal" part of adolescence. The increase in fatigue between childhood and adolescence almost certainly reflects both the physiological demands of growth and dramatic increases in social and educational demands. Two thirds of adolescents report morning fatigue to the extent of impairing their waking more than once a week.

Acute fatigue syndromes associated with viral illnesses are very common among teenagers. These states are particularly marked with certain viral infections, such as Epstein-Barr virus infections (mononucleosis or glandular fever). In developed countries, Epstein-Barr virus is predominantly an illness of teenagers and few reach their 20s without seroconversion; about 9% are estimated to develop severe acute fatigue syndrome after infection. Treatment of such postviral acute fatigue syndrome consists of excluding secondary bacterial infection or anaemia and providing reassurance.

### Chronic fatigue syndrome

Fatigue in young people is serious when it persists for more than three months and impairs school attendance, academic results, and peer relationships. The definition of chronic fatigue syndrome (CFS) in adults has been much debated. The syndrome, often known by patients as myalgic encephalomyelitis or postviral fatigue syndrome, was first commonly described in the 1980s and is now claimed by some researchers to be the commonest medical cause of long term absence from school. Recent epidemiological evidence suggests that chronic fatigue syndrome, as defined on the basis of the criteria of the Centers for Disease Control and Prevention (CDC), occurs in about 0.2-0.6% of adolescents aged 11-15 years.

Continuing controversy over the existence of CFS, together with uncertainty and contradictory research findings about aetiology and treatment, has made the management of CFS extremely difficult for health professionals and patients alike. In Britain, this situation recently led to a report by the chief medical officer that acknowledged the reality of the illness in children and young people and emphasised that good quality, evidence based care should be provided.

The aetiology of CFS is unknown, with many hypotheses proposed. No convincing evidence exists to support persisting viral infection. Patients do show an excess of depression, other psychological symptoms, and low self esteem, although data on the psychological and endocrine states of patients show that CFS is not merely a masked form of depression, somatoform disorder, or refusal to attend school. Given the high prevalence of acute postviral fatigue syndromes in adolescence, it is unclear why acute fatigue syndromes become chronic in some young

---

### Differential diagnosis of chronic abdominal pain

*Common causes*—Functional abdominal pain, constipation, dysmenorrhoea, urinary tract infection, dyspepsia associated with *Helicobacter pylori*, irritable bowel syndrome
*Uncommon causes*—Chronic appendicitis, pelvic inflammatory disease, gastro-oesophageal reflux, peptic ulcer disease, mittelschmerz
*Rare causes*—Inflammatory bowel disease, renal calculi, ovarian cyst, biliary calculi, sickle cell crisis

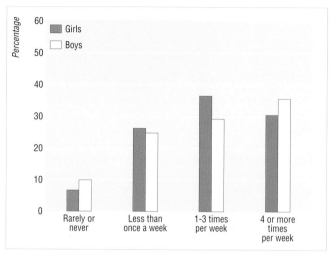

Frequency of serious morning fatigue in 11-17 year olds in Europe. Adapted from *Health behaviour in school-aged children, 1997-1998* (see first graph)

---

### Centers for Disease Control and Prevention's diagnostic criteria for chronic fatigue syndrome*

#### Major criteria (both required)
- Debilitating fatigue reducing activity to less than 50% of the patient's premorbid activity for at least six months (in practice, with adolescents this is usually reduced to three months)
- Symptoms not explained by other medical or chronic psychiatric illness

*The presence of non-psychotic depression does not preclude the diagnosis of chronic fatigue syndrome*

#### Symptom criteria (four required)
- Sore throat
- Painful cervical or axillary lymphadenopathy
- Muscle discomfort or pain
- Prolonged generalised fatigue after usual levels of activity
- Headaches
- Arthralgias (without swelling or redness)
- Neuropsychological disorders such as forgetfulness and lack of concentration
- Sleep disturbance (unrefreshing sleep)

*Adapted from Fukuda et al. The chronic fatigue syndrome: a comprehensive approach to its definition and study. *Ann Intern Med* 1994;121:953-9.

---

### Key points from chief medical officer's working party on chronic fatigue syndrome for young people

- Young people do develop CFS, although many recover
- Important differences exist between children and adults in the nature and impact of the syndrome and its management
- CFS can threaten adolescents' physical, emotional, and intellectual development and disrupt education and social and family life
- A prompt and authoritative diagnosis is needed
- Ideal management is patient centred, community based, multidisciplinary, and coordinated, with regular follow up
- Community paediatric services need to be available for most young people and all those with prolonged school absence
- The clinician who coordinates care must consider early the educational needs and impact on the family and parents (or carers)

people. One study among adults has suggested that major events and depression around the time of Epstein-Barr virus infection may be linked to the persistence of fatigue.

CFS is likely to be a collection of different conditions and that several biopsychosocial "causal pathways" can lead to chronic fatigue. It is therefore best understood as a chronic low functioning state in which biological causal factors have resolved yet the illness remains because of physical deconditioning, sleep disturbance, and psychosocial factors. In adolescence, CFS usually occurs soon after the transition from primary to secondary school (onset peaks at 12-14 years). This is a time when young people are exposed, through mixing in larger schools, to new infections (such as Epstein-Barr virus) and to considerable stresses from the greater demands of secondary school. Rest and withdrawal from school and normal activities can lead to frustration, alternating overactivity and underactivity, disturbed sleep, social isolation, and depression, all of which may help to maintain the chronic fatigue.

Patients must be assessed with a combined biopsychosocial approach (once treatable conditions have been excluded). The differential diagnosis includes endocrine abnormalities, connective tissue disorders, neurological disorders, and psychological disorders (including depression, eating disorders, and refusal syndromes). Psychosocial assessment should include consideration of individual and family function; relationships with friends; school performance; and history of bullying, refusal to attend school, and psychiatric disorders. The most common comorbid psychological problems include depression and sleep disturbance.

CFS in young people should be diagnosed promptly and authoritatively and not be a delayed diagnosis of exclusion. Published case series suggest that most young people are substantially better or cured within two to three years.

# Management of fatigue and somatic symptoms

After treatable causes of persistent somatic symptoms have been excluded, management based on a rehabilitative model is helpful for most young people. However, it is essential not to label symptoms as psychological, as this will often alienate the family. Some families readily understand the nature of psychosomatic causation, but many young people and their families are resistant to a psychological explanation for the symptoms and feel that such explanations mean they are not being believed.

It is generally more helpful to avoid such simplistic mind-body splits and avoid searching for psychological problems or "causes" within the family. But acknowledge such problems where they are apparent.

It is most useful to take a two pronged pragmatic approach, based on improving function while controlling symptoms. With a pragmatic approach, families generally accept the importance of psychological factors if it is recognised that these factors may equally be consequences as much as causes of illness. Rehabilitation involving physical, psychological, and social elements can be useful in chronic pain or chronic fatigue syndromes.

## Chronic fatigue syndrome

Randomised clinical trials in adults have shown that cognitive behaviour therapy and graded exercise programmes are helpful in most patients. Uncontrolled studies in young people suggest that outpatient multidisciplinary rehabilitation and cognitive behaviour therapy within the family are helpful. An individual

**Common additional features of chronic fatigue syndrome in adolescents**

- Abdominal pains
- Nausea
- Loss of appetite
- Weight loss or failure to gain weight appropriately for age
- Blurred vision
- Fall in school performance and attendance

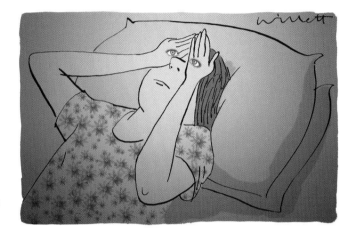

**Medical investigations for chronic fatigue syndrome***

- Full blood count
- Acute phase protein changes (erythrocyte sedimentation rate, C reactive protein)
- Basic biochemistry tests
- Thyroid function
- Creatine kinase testing
- Immunoglobulin testing
- Autoantibody screen (including antinuclear antibodies, rheumatoid factor, coeliac antibodies)
- More extensive investigations (testing for glucocorticoid deficiency and viral serology— for example, for Epstein-Barr virus and Lyme disease—if indicated by history or symptoms)

*Adapted from *Chronic Fatigue Syndrome* (see Further Reading box)

**Managing complex somatic symptoms**

- Acknowledge the reality of symptoms despite a lack of known cause
- Avoid simplistic mind-body splits
- Enable ownership of the management programme by the young person; engagement of the patient and family is essential
- Focus on functional improvement through rehabilitation and on symptom control
- Use multidisciplinary approaches; occupational therapy can be particularly helpful
- Engage the patient in setting goals, with frequent reviews

**Generic rehabilitation programme for teenagers**

- Graded "return to school" programme, combined with home tuition
- Activities and exercise programme, graded over many months and supervised by physiotherapist or occupational therapist
- Family support—informal or with formal family therapy sessions
- Cognitive behaviour therapy

**No high quality evidence exists to guide the treatment of chronic fatigue syndrome in children and young people**

programme should be developed for each patient, based on the identification of maintenance factors that prevent recovery: biological factors (such as sleep disturbance and physical deconditioning); psychological factors (such as personality, coping style, and comorbid depression); and social factors (such as family losses or stress, or parental conflict over management of their child's condition).

## Chronic pain

Management of recurrent or persistent pain can be extremely difficult. When symptoms are severe, persistent, and unexplained, it may help to consider the problem as a regional chronic pain syndrome. This focuses the management on chronic pain as a symptom rather than on finding a cause related to the specific site of the pain. Lack of exacerbating and relieving factors and lack of response to analgesia are common characteristics of chronic pain syndromes. The most effective treatment for such syndromes in young people is multidisciplinary rehabilitation alongside symptom control. Although this can be done in primary care, the involvement of a chronic pain service with experience of adolescents can be extremely useful.

---

**Management of chronic fatigue syndrome**

- Rehabilitation should be multidisciplinary
- Selective serotonin reuptake inhibitors may raise energy levels if mood is low, but no evidence exists of effectiveness
- Melatonin may be helpful if sleep is badly disturbed, but no evidence exists of effectiveness
- Inpatient rehabilitation is rarely necessary; use only if outpatient management fails

---

**Further reading and resources**

- NHS Centre for Reviews and Dissemination. Interventions for the management of CFS/ME. *Effective Health Care* 2002;7:1-12
- CFS/ME Working Group. Report of the CFS/ME working group: report to the chief medical officer of an independent working group. 2002. (Search via www.dh.gov.uk)
- Royal College of Physicians. *Chronic fatigue syndrome*. London: RCP, 1996. (Report of a joint working group of the Royal Colleges of Physicians, Psychiatrists and General Practitioners.)
- McGregor RS. Chronic complaints in adolescence: chest pain, chronic fatigue, headaches, abdominal pain. *Adolescent Medicine State of the Art Reviews* 1997;8:15-31.
- www.ayme.org.uk (Action for Youth with ME is a useful and effective patient support group)

---

**Management of chronic pain**

- Rehabilitation should be multidisciplinary
- Amitryptyline and fluoxetine in moderate doses may help to reduce pain, promote sleep, and lift mood, regardless of the presence of depression
- Hypnotherapy may be helpful
- Other complementary therapies—such as massage or aromatherapy—may help
- Consultation with a chronic pain service is useful when the treatment above does not control symptoms or improve function. Drugs such as gabapentin should be used only in a chronic pain service

# Index

*Notes*: Page numbers in *italics* refer to figures and tables.

# Index

# Index